HEAVY METALS. THE WHITE SABBATH OF TOXINS

RICHARD C. SEMELKA

HEAVY METALS. THE WHITE SABBATH OF TOXINS

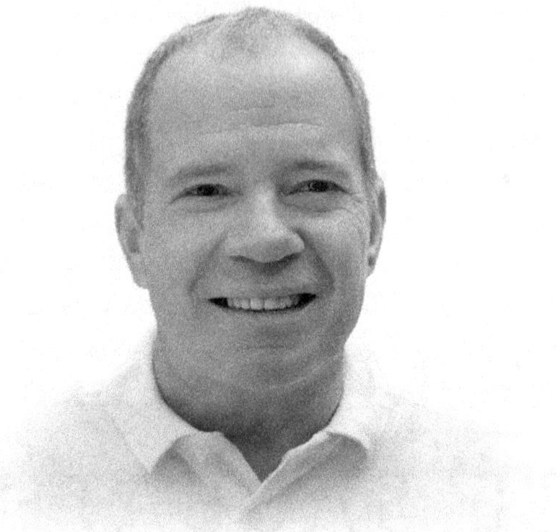

HEAVY METALS

The White Sabbath of Toxins

This book is intended for members of the public who are informed about health care matters. It is written in a concise, comprehensible fashion, and focuses on key aspects of heavy metal toxicity, who gets it, what are the symptoma, what is the best current treatment, and what is the outcome, Special emphasis is placed on providing the most up-to-date treatment regimens for heavy metal toxicity.

ABOUT THE AUTHOR

ScholarGPS has rated my career in the top 0.05% of all scholars in all fields. For 35 years, I've worked with, and been one of the leading authors on, gadolinium-based contrast agents (GBCAs) used in MRis, which are heavy metals bound to chelators. I've written over 300 peer-reviewed papers and six major textbooks focused on both the value of GBCAs and their toxicities, including gadolinium deposition disease (GDD), Over the last nine years. I have become the world authority on the dlagnosis and treatment of heavy metal toxicity, primarily gadolinium, but also lead, mercury and others. Patients come to my clinic from around the world based on my established expertise.

CONTENTS

HEAVY METALS

The White Sabbath of Toxins

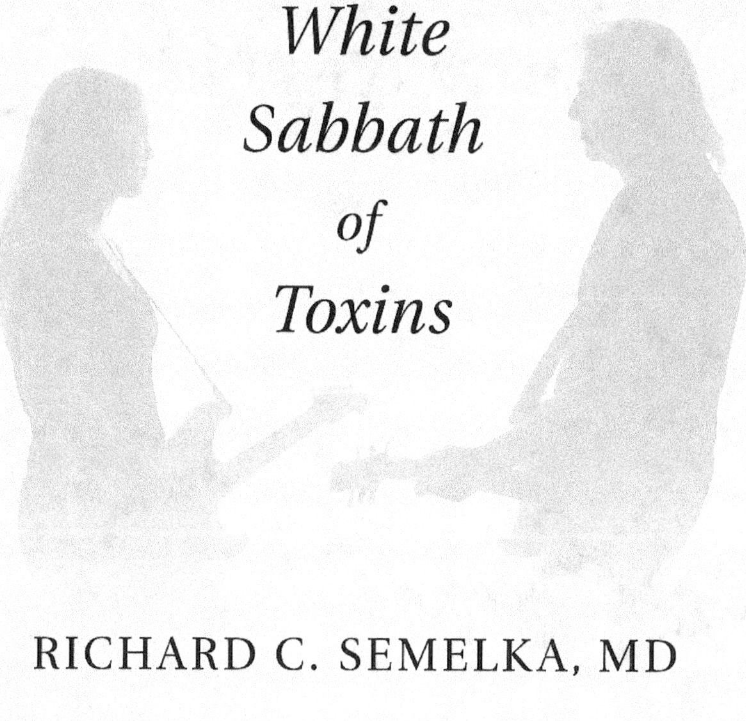

RICHARD C. SEMELKA, MD

CHAPTER

One

HEAVY METALS IN THE CONTEXT OF TOXINS.

Chapter 1. Heavy Metals in the context of toxins.

Toxins by definition are agents that can cause harm to living organisms, generally by disrupting biological processes or damaging tissues and cells. The term host will be used frequently throughout this book to refer to the living organism, and the host that is focused on is humans. Toxins can be grouped into two large categories: chemical and biological. Chemical toxins include: heavy metals, microplastics, PFAS, glyphosates; and biological toxins include viruses, bacteria, mold, Lyme Disease, and I include vaccine-caused toxicity in this latter category.

These chemical toxins show increasing environmental toxicity. Boahen and co-authors have written an excellent review describing the categories of: micro- and nanoplastics (MNPs), PFAS, pharmaceuticals and personal care products (PPCPs), endocrine-disrupting chemicals (EDCs), and persistent organic pollutants (POPs). Microplastics deserve special mention in the context of heavy metal toxins, as investigators have shown that heavy metals can adhere to the surface of microplastics. Therefore microplastics may serve to both increase the amount of heavy metal deposition but also potentially make that deposition more durable.

Within the category of chemical toxins, heavy metals are unique in that treatment does not entail breaking down the agent, because metal atoms cannot be broken down. Hence treatment is focused on removal of the agents. Most chemical toxins likely represent forever chemicals. PFAS are the typical chemical group bearing this designation. The human toxicity/ damage caused by many of these are presently unknown, but obviously must exist. Heavy metals behave as forever chemicals, as most of the ones described in this book can bind to tissues and remain there.

The ability to remove heavy metals, described below, does separate heavy metals from the others. Detoxification represents the modification of either the toxin or the hosts own defenses to render the substance less injurious. Modifying the host defenses achieves the goal of improving/amplifying metabolic activity against the agent. Detoxification therefore generally entails some form of degradation of the toxin. The general concept of strengthening the host's defenses is an invariable part of combating all toxins, including heavy metals. Because of the durable, immutable nature of the atoms of stable heavy metals this does lend these toxins to the definitive type of removal treatment, which is chelation. Chelation basically represents molecules grabbing the metal atoms, and holding on to them to result in removal. The strength of the grabbing and holding on to heavy metals is termed the stability or affinity, and in scientific terms shown by the log stability constant. This will be referred to throughout this book, as it is of crucial importance.

Radioactive metals which decay with release of radiation energy, still end up as lower atomic number metals. Of all the chemical toxins that afflict humans, heavy metals are the one category that can potentially experience near or effective cure,because they can be removed, and hence the root cause treated. This effective cure is mediated by chelation.

This text will describe the optimal currently available chelation methods for heavy metals, and the best available approaches, even if they are not yet widely used. The fact that some approaches are not yet widely used does not reflect that the approaches described herein are in some fashion experimental, but rather that the community of health care workers are not fully informed in a full knowledge of heavy metals and the science of treatment. This book serves to address that. I will also describe which heavy metals still require significant improvement of treatment and explain why. This text is not intending to be an exhaustive approach to chelation, and will not include less effective chelators, so that there is no risk of the reader misinterpreting that poorer strategies are advocated. Heavy metals result in Immune Mediated Inflammatory Disease (IMIDs), and these can act together with other IMIDs to contribute to global Immune System Dysregulation (ISD). This will be a recurring theme throughout this text, emphasizing its critical importance.

Further reading:

1.Boahen, E., Franklin, S., & May, A. (2025). A comprehensive review of emerging
environmental contaminants: occurrence, fate, and potential impacts. Environmental
Science and Pollution Research. https://doi.org/10.1007/

s44274-025-00259-x
2. McInnes, I. B., & Gravallese, E. M.. Immune-mediated inflammatory disease
therapeutics. 2021. Nature Reviews Immunology. 21: 548–564.
3. Long, A. Immune dysregulation. 2023. Journal of Allergy and Clinical Immunology
(Review).152: 1088-1102.
4. Monteleone, G., Pallone, F., & Stolfi, C. X. Immune-mediated inflammatory diseases:
Common and divergent pathways. Best Practice & Research Clinical Gastroenterology.
22: article 103410.
5. Schett, G., McInnes, I. B., & Neurath, M. F. 2021) Reframing immune-mediated
inflammatory diseases through signature cytokine hubs."New England Journal of
Medicine, 385, 628-639.
6. Baker K F, et al. Biomarkers of tolerance in immune-mediated inflammatory diseases.
2021. The Lancet Rheumatology.3: e371-e382.
7. Mahalingiah S, Nadeau KC, Christiani DC. Microplastics in human health.

CHAPTER

Two

EXPOSURE SOURCES OF HEAVY METALS

Chapter 2. Exposure Sources of Heavy Metals.

The element symbols most often reflect the modern English language name of the metal. A quirk of the element symbols in the Periodic table are metIn the majority of cases, exposure sources of heavy metals are secondary to human activity, and the creation of various forms of pollution in the environment. The morepolluted the regional environment of the host individual, the more likely they will be to acquire heavy metal toxins.A generic panel of potentially toxic heavy metals that are tested for by commercial labs include the following metals with metal element symbol in parentheses that have been identified in antiquity and have a Latin name, the symbol is based on that, which includes: Antimony (Sb), Lead (Pb), Mercury (Hg) and Tin (Sn).Aluminum (Al), Antimony (Sb), Arsenic (As), Barium (Ba), Beryllium (Be), Bismuth (Bi),Cadmium (Cd), Cesium (Cs), Gadolinium (Gd), Lead (Pb), Mercury (Hg), Nickel

(Ni),Palladium (Pd), Platinum (Pt), Tellurium (Te), Thallium (Tl), Thorium (Th), Tin (Sn), Tungsten (W), Uranium (U).

Rare Earth metals are heavy metals in the Lanthinide series, which are a group of 15 metals in the periodic table that start with Lanthanum and end with Lutetium. Gadolinium is within the Rare Earth group of metals. Rare Earth metals have similar properties and are generally used in the construction of magnets and electronics. Lanthanum carbonate is used as a phosphate binder in the gut in patients on renal dialysis. It is orally administered and often given as chewable tablets with meals. Lanthanum is not part of the standard toxic metal panel of metals, so its actual adverse health impact is untested and hence unknown. Lanthanum probably should be included in standard panels because of its use in medical human application.

The next series of metals, which are heavier in atomic number, are the Actinide metals, many of which are radioactive. Plutonium and Uranium are in this series. Radioactive metals have their own additional toxicity which results from release of high energy particles in the process of the element undergoing radioactive decay. Radioactive metals most often decay to a lower atomic number heavy metal, so the decayed product is still a heavy metal. Radioactive metals are used for their radioactive properties, and are utilized in medical applications, nuclear reactors and other nuclear applications. Plutonium is often not measured in standard panels.

Many of the chapters in this book are dedicated to specific heavy metals, and the more detailed description of sources will be described therein. Clinical history obtained
from patients with suspected heavy metal toxicity will require inquiry into: employment history, such as military, battery factory worker, nuclear plant worker, electronic
manufacture worker; lead exposure from municipal water; diet/ food consumption; and prior MRI with a Gadolinium Based Con-

trast Agent (GBCA). Although most heavy metals share similar symptoms, there are some symptoms that are distinctive for certain metals, and will be discussed in the relevant chapter of those metals.

Further Reading:

1. Li M., Hu J., Zhang Z. Heavy Metal Contamination: Sources, Health Impacts, and Mitigation. International Journal of Environmental Research and Public Health. 2024. 21(3), 2351-2365.
This review covers heavy metal sources, pathways, toxicological impacts, and mitigation strategies.
2. Zhao F-J, Jiang R-F, Dunham S J, McGrath S P.. A Review on Heavy Metals Contamination in Soil: Effects, Sources, and Remediation Technologies. 2019. Journal of Soil Contamination & Remediation; 19(6), 1-22.
This one discusses various sources of heavy metals in soils (natural weathering, mining, smelting, agrochemicals, industrial emissions) and remediation methods.

CHAPTER

Three

GENERIC SYMPTOMS OF TOXICITY

Chapter 3. Generic Symptoms of Heavy Metal Toxicity.

Deposition Disease and Storage Condition States.
Acute Exposure. Chronic Exposure. Generic Symptoms.
Heavy metal toxicities can result in a wide range of symptoms throughout the body. This is because most heavy metals distribute throughout the body, and a broad range of symptoms occur from diseases that are systemic. There are a few types and patterns of symptoms that are fairly common that are shared by nearly all heavy metal toxicities. These include:

Central neurological symptoms
Cognitive impairment.
Peripheral neurological symptoms.
Numbness and tingling in the hands and feet.
Fatigue
Headache
Digestive System symptoms: nausea and abdominal pain

Kidney damage: decreased renal function

Skin: rashes and discoloration.

Individual heavy metals can result in distinctive symptoms, and these will be discussed in chapters dedicated to those metals.

The above generic symptoms for heavy metals include a cluster of symptoms that are also common for infectious diseases, especially viral diseases. A critical distinction between Heavy Metal Toxicity and diffuse disease from Infective organisms (viruses, bacteria, fungi) is that heavy metal toxicity rarely results in fever, and certainly not significantly elevated temperature, whereas infective organisms almost always do. Absence of fever in an individual with systemic symptoms of cognitive impairment, headache, fatigue, abdominal pain, fits with the possibility of a heavy metal toxicity as a cause for disease, and mitigates against infection. Infections also are generally associated with an elevation of neutrophils, the group of immune cells that generally respond to infection, and heavy metals do not have this effect.

Toxicity. Deposition Disease State and Storage Condition State. Essentially everyone has lead in their body. Also essentially everyone has at least 3heavy metals (often 5 or more) in their body, that can be most easily revealed with native (also termed unprovoked) 24 hour urine study. It is important to note that this does not mean that they are sick from those heavy metals, which is to say that they are not experiencing toxicity. A specific term for the presence of a heavy metal in the body without evidence of toxicity is Storage Condition. The circumstance in which the individual is experiencing significant symptoms from the presence of a heavy metal, traditionally termed toxicity, the more specific term that describes that the individual has both the heavy metal retained in their body and are sick from it is Deposition DIsease.

Acute and Chronic Symptoms and Exposures.

In general retention of heavy metals that is causing sickness in the individual, a transition gradually occurs from acute toxicity symptoms/findings to chronic. Inapproximate terms this transition occurs in the 1 month time frame. Exposures can be acute or chronic in type. An MRI study Gadolinium Based Contrast Agent (GBCA) injection is an example of an acute exposure. Most heavymetals are acquired in a more protracted fashion, as they reflect ongoing exposure, and this represents chronic exposure. The distinction of describing a heavy metal toxicity exposure as Acute is important when the dose received is massive. This is described by the observation attributed to Paracelsus: the dose makes the poison (in Latin: Dosis sola facit venenum).

Classic examples for the prominence of Acute exposure is when the heavy metal has a particularly high toxicity severity index: such as Arsenic poisoning, or when the heavy metal is radioactive, such as Plutonium. For this latter category of radioactive metals it is the toxicity of the radioactive decay of the atoms with release of high energy atomic and subatomic particles that causes the extreme damage, not the less direct tissue destructive interference and blockade of metabolic function that stable heavy metals

cause.

For most heavy metals, the exposure generally is somewhat insidious and reflects ongoing long term exposure, typical for Lead, Cadmium and Chromium. So distinct acute phases and chronic phases are not clearly defined. As Gadolinium (Gd) is incorporated as an abrupt short term exposure, performed as iv administration of a GBCA, acute and chronic symptoms can be more clearly defined.

Extrapolation from Gd to other heavy metals can be made for distinction of acute and chronic symptoms. Acute toxicity symptoms from Gd are oftentimes observed as progressive development of additional symptoms over the course of 1 to several weeks. So this may be observed as initial headache and cognitive impairment from immediate to within 1 day post-injection, progressing to muscle twitching, skin pain, bone pain over a course of 1-4 weeks as acute toxicity symptoms Late chronic symptoms generally commence at 3 months, with typical findings: hair loss, skin thickening, loss of soft tissue. So acute symptoms generally arise within 1 month and chronic symptoms start to appear at 3 months. The acute symptoms generally reflect the effect of vascular transport of pro-inflammatory cytokines and other inflammatory cell products, and other immediate cellular actions such as dysregulating cell membrane transport functions. The chronic symptoms reflect progressive tissue production, generally fibrosis (scarring), and destruction (tissue loss) changes. All these changes vary considerably between individuals. There is not a set pattern that defines which acute symptoms develop first nor how they progress. Nor do all individuals with longstanding disease develop chronic symptoms or findings. At present these appear to occur somewhat unpredictably, withthe exception that headache is a very common initial symptom. This variability is not random, but reflects a complex interplay between immunologic and toxic effects of metals, and an enormous range of potential host responses.

An additional reaction observed with Gd, which may not occur with other heavy metals, is acute hypersensitivity reaction (AHR) that can result in a cytokine storm and rarely in severe anaphylactoid reaction, that can cause immediate death. Gd is uniquely experienced as an abrupt and forceful high velocity systemic exposure by intravenous injection, that none of the other heavy metals entail. The transition from AHR to Gadolinium Deposition Disease (GDD), likely reflects the transition of the type of dominant immune cells engaged in the host response. Very early response is by MASTcell dominant reaction, the cell type that causes AHR, that occurs from immediate to 2-3days, and this transitions to tissue resident memory T cell dominant reaction at 2-4 days. Our current theory is 'pure' GDD arises at 2-4 days. This will be discussed in greater detail in the Gadolinium chapter.

Many of the heavy metal exposures are a long term ongoing process, often insidious and initially imperceptible. Most usually arise from toxic environmental exposure, such as from contaminated water (lead, chromium), or initiated as air pollution that transfers to soil and either acquired in humans as soil or as living entities grown in soil (Thallium,Cesium) such as kale. More dramatic is insidious or acute exposure performed nefariously, famously Arsenic and Thallium. Although highly memorable, these intentional true poisonings are thankfully rare. Nonetheless massive acute exposures may occur with any heavy metal, and often in these settings the presentation is with massive neurological symptoms such as seizures. The outcomes for these massive exposures are usually very dismal. The relative frequency of a Heavy Metal Storage Condition compared to Heavy Metal Deposition Disease is in the order of 10,000 to 1 for Gd, which also appears to be the same ratio with lead. Our theory is this ratio is likely also present for other heavy metals. Our opinion is that the dose for most of the metals does change the ratio. The higher the dose the more likely the individual will experience toxicity: Deposition Disease. It bears emphasizing that it is likely the immunologic response of the host that is crucial to either allowing or preventing disease.

These exact mechanisms are now the subject of ongoing research, as will be described in the chapter on Future Directions.

Further Reading:.

1.Semelka RC, Ramalho M. Gadolinium Toxicity and Current State of Knowledge and
Expert Opinion. Investigative Radiology 2023; 58: 233-245

2. Johnson TA, Nguyen LP. .Autoimmunity-Induced Neurotoxicity from Heavy Metals. J
Autoimmunity Research 2025; 34: 102-115.

3. Bjorklund G, Buha Dordevic A, Hamdan H, Wallace DR, Peana M. Metal-
Induced Autoimmunity in Neurological Disorders: A View of Current
Understanding and Future Directions. Autoimmunity Reviews 2024; 23: article
103509.

CHAPTER

Four

WHO ARE AT RISK?

Chapter 4. Who are at risk? Increased exposure/ increased susceptibility.

Increased Exposure

As a general rule, the adage of Paracelsus **'the dose makes the poison'**, is true for heavy metals, as it is for most things. So, the greater the exposure, either as a single administration or multiple/continuous exposure, the greater the likelihood of and the greater the severity of toxicity. The initial and primary form of management is avoidance, usually this means minimization of exposure as it is virtually impossible to avoid environmental heavy metal toxins from pollution.

Individuals who work with heavy metals such as vehicle assembly line workers, welders, electronics, battery manufacture, have a greater exposure to many types of heavy metals than the average person.

Some of the most recognized increased exposures are from sites of chemical dumping. Perhaps the most famous reporter being Erin Brokovich, who described a large contamination location of chromium. Another important group is individuals in the southwest USA living in areas close to where nuclear testing was done in the 1950s, resulting in high Uranium levels.

The greatest effort for the minimization of a heavy metal exposure has been, and continues to be, with lead. In the 1970s legislation for lead removal from gasoline was progressively introduced. Lead was mandated to be removed from paint in the 1960s. In the current 2020s nationwide effort to remove lead from plumbing pipes is underway. Nonetheless lead continues to be discovered in all sorts of products that may readily incorporate into our bodies. Baby food, tampons, and very recently various processed foods, are just a few examples. An unknown amount of lead is also transferred to the growing fetus through maternal-fetal circulation that occurs at the placenta.

Another example of ongoing attention to toxins, and subsequent elimination of some pathways of heavy metal exposure, was the elimination of Arsenic from chicken feed in the mid 1990s.

The above are examples of government--mediated decreases in heavy metal exposures. Corporation-driven reductions in exposure have been critical for decrease in Mercury from contaminated fish, and Cadmium from rice and shellfish. Individual consumer driven changes include reduction in Thallium and Cesium by reduced consumption of kale. For the future, consumer-driven changes may be essential for quick recognition of high heavy metal presence in products, and minimizing their use, or consumer advocacy driving change in companies, for example lead content in baby food.

Increased Susceptibility

There are a variety of genetic, epigenetic, environmental, immunological and intrinsic health status that affects how susceptible an individual is to heavy metal toxicity/ deposition disease.

A short background on genetics: Genes represent DNA sequence pairs on chromosomes that provide the code to build proteins. Proteins accomplish essentially all functions in the body, Genes vary in length from hundreds of DNA pairs to in the millions. So genetics is a major driving force in all physiology in our bodies, and they code the proteins which are basically the worker bees for every function.

The most recognized genetic cause for a metal toxicity is Genetic Hemochromatosis (GH), that results from an abnormal imbalanced increased absorption of Iron in the digestive tract, which leads to iron overload.. The clinical findings of greatest importance in GH are: pancreas deposition, liver deposition, heart deposition and bone deposition. GH is described more fully in an upcoming chapter. The gene that is the most common cause of GH is the HFE gene, and the most frequent mutation to cause disease is C282Y.

Epigenetic refers to the circumstance where the genes that are formed by DNA sequencing are not altered, but the expression of these genes are modified. So modifications include turning on or off, or increasing (upregulating) or decreasing (downregulating) the activity of the genes. These modifications can be induced by numerous factors including environment and lifestyle.

In my opinion, the majority of heavy metal toxicities are due to genetic and/or epigenetic causes, which are at present not elucidated.

Different gender/ racial susceptibilities to heavy metal toxicities are observed. For example GH is observed almost exclusively in individuals with European genetics of central (Gaulic/ French) origin.

Gadolinium toxicity/ deposition disease most commonly arises in white females, a predisposition that is common for autoimmune diseases in general.

This will be discussed in greater detail in upcoming chapters.

Further Reading:

1. Lanphear B. Lead Poisoning. New England Journal of Medicine 2024; 390: 501-513.

2. Semelka RC, Ramalho M. Gadolinium Toxicity and Current State of Knowledge and

Expert Opinion. Investigative Radiology 2023; 58: 233-245.

3. Bagni G. Epigenetics in Autoimmune Diseases: Unraveling the Complexities. Clinical Epigenetics 2025; 17: 87-102.

CHAPTER

Five

IMMUNE MEDIATED INFLAMMATORY DISEASE

Chapter 5. Immune Mediated Inflammatory Disease. Immune System Dysregulation. Composite immune mediated inflammatory disease and toxicity. The web of interconnected entities and processes in health and disease.

The appreciation of the interconnections in the human biological system has been a subject of intense interest over the last decade. The understanding of the interplay between normal organs and tissues, interconnections of disease in one organ system affecting other distant organ systems, for example digestive tract disease creating abnormalities in the skin and central nervous system. Most recently, interconnections between various disease entities with other disease states, their effect on proteins and cytokines, and where the same entities may behave differently in different environments. In short, everything in the body has an effect on everything else in the body, and the key to management is to achieve a balance between all sources to result in the best possible state of health, despite everything that is going on. In other words,focus on the Goldilocks principle. Heavy metals toxicity are excellent examples of this interconnection. Toxicity developing to 1 heavy metal often results in the susceptibility to other heavy metals. In the broadest sense, heavy metals that become toxic have induced an Immune Mediated Inflammatory Disease (IMID) as a precursor to causing direct toxicity in many cases. The IMID to a heavy metal can arise from, or result in, IMIDs to other agents that can cause immunological reaction. Common entities include infective agents (COVID, Lyme, Epstein Barr, Cytomegalovirus, Herpes), vaccines, PFAs, glyphosates, mold, as a partial list. I use the Latin expression to reflect this relationship: Abyssuss Abyssum Invocat. (One hell calls forth another).What is noteworthy, is that different families of IMID are more or less likely to cause heavy metal IMID, and thereby toxicity. It appears that IMIDs that have an effect on the total body (systemic) have a much greater propensity to activate IMID from heavy metals, which are also systemic. So long COVID which is a systemic disease has a much greater likelihood of creating susceptibility to Gadolinium toxicity, than does asthma, which is a lung regional IMID.

The complexity of the Immune system. Its focus is on achieving balance:

The concept emphasized in this text of the crucial role of the immune system in heavy metal toxicities, actually is in concert with the 2025 Nobel Prize in Medicine and Science for the description of T regulatory cells or Tregs. I emphasize in this book the concept of Immune System Dysregulation (ISD).

To provide a succinct evaluation of this concept. There are 3 basic categories of T cells: T effector (T eff) cells with subcategory helper cells (Th); T regulatory cells (T regs); and a third category, that I term T communicating cells (Tcom). In general terms the principal activity of these categories are: T eff cells are pro-inflammatory; T regs are anti-inflammatory (immune reaction dampening); and T com inform the cells in the body how to behave. The important understanding is that to maintain health in the entire body, there has to be an overall balance between these cell populations and cell functions. Often it is not a pure numbers game when a person is in an inflammatory state, so the only abnormality is not more T Helper cells, but that the overall balance reflecting the number, level of activation and level of function of T Helper cells is greater than the number, level of activation, and level of function of T regs.

Next in importance is to look at the cytokines, there are: proinflammatory cytokines, anti-inflammatory cytokines, and communicating cytokines.

Immune dampening cytokines:

1. Transforming growth factor Beta (TGF- Beta)
2. Interleukin-10 (IL-10).

Pro-inflammatory cytokines:

1. Tumor necrosis factor- Alpha (TNF-Alpha)
2. IL-1 Beta
3. IL-5 (more specialized stimulates growth and activation of eosinophils)
4. IL-6
5. IL-17A
6. Interferon -gamma

The picture is much more complicated than Th cells release only pro-inflammatory cytokines and T reg cells release only anti-inflammatory cytokines (immune reaction dampening). All Tcells can release many different types of cytokines, it is the overall balance of what they release that has the dominant effect. With Th cells the balance of cytokines is pro-inflammatory. Similarly, with Tregs the balance is immune reaction dampening. Furthermore an additional twist is that in different combinations and different milieus cytokines of one type can behave like another, so pro-inflammatory cytokines can behave as immune dampening.

The third category of T cells, T communicating, behave more as messengers, and basically message other cells to maintain homeostasis. For example in the presence of Gadolinium or Lead in the system, in the normal, non-reacting setting, they would communicate to cells to stay calm and not to overreact. There are also different subpopulations of these cells, so there are Th1, Th2, and Th17 as an example.

The category of T cells that I emphasize as a major driver in heavy metal toxicity are Tissue resident Memory T cells. These can be a mixture of Th and Treg cells. These are the dominant cells causing disease in autoimmune conditions such as Rheumatoid Arthritis and Crohn's. In individuals with Heavy Metal Deposition Disease/ toxicity the balance of function would be towards pro-inflammation Th cells. There may or may not be more Th cells, but it is that the overall effect is pro-inflammation.

The complexity inherent in the inflammatory picture does emphasize the critical and central importance of chelation removal of the heavy metal. The immune picture can be so complex in an Immune System Dysregulation, that any particular intervention that empirically may achieve immune dampening, may instead result in the opposite effect. This should not be misconstrued that the immune system is so complex that one has to neglect it, but rather to recognize its importance and its potential for variability of reaction. Therefore one has to be cautious with interventions.

Timelines in Immunity:

There are a number of physiological reactions for different processes that serve as surrogates for understanding development of HeavyMetal Toxicity / Deposition Disease.

One of these is appreciating 3 landmarks of immunity development and tissue response to injury: 1) full immunity to viral vaccines are generally understood to occur at around 14 days, so 14 days serves as a time point when an IMID reaction to a heavy metal becomes at full force; 2) development of substantial granulation tissue, which is immature, vascularized precursor to fibrosis, occurs generally by 3 months. This process occurs for many significant immune reactions, which includes post-surgery, post-radiation and Heavy Metal Toxicity. Granulation tissue is still at an early stage, so it is readily reversible; and 3) development of mature fibrosis is established by 1 year.Mature fibrosis is much less treatable. These 3 time points provide target dates when certain treatment approaches can be employed.

Chelation prior to 2 weeks is at a time that full immune reaction has not developed, so rigorous concurrent steroid treatment may not be necessary, and significant elimination of heavy metal can be achieved. At 3 months substantial cellular reaction to a toxin has begun to develop (granulation tissue is one of the core reactions) and this frequently can be reversed, so chelation starting at 3 months in general is quite ideal. By one year the response has become more mature, treatment is then more challenging and will take more sessions of chelation. Cure is still achievable even years after the disease has started though, but is generally not complete. Chelation is explained in more detail in an upcoming chapter.

Another useful comparison to understand the elements of chelation is how all healing occurs, for example of the skin. Healing is performed in 3 phases: 1) early destruction (0-2 days), 2) creation of granulation tissue for healing (1-7 days), and 3) remodeling (7 days - 3 months).These are average time points in the healthy condition. An important understanding is that these 3 processes all occur at the same time, it is the relative proportion of the activity that varies over time. This can be thought of as a carefully choreographed symphony. This is essentially the same process that occurs with chelation: 1) early removal of the metal from less tightly bound tissue reservoirs, 2) stabilization with evidence of improvement, and 3) movement of heavy metal from most tightly bound locations back to the more loosely bound locations, from which most of the metal was removed. Considering the bone-deposting metals of Gadolinium, Lead and Cadmium as examples: 1) Heavy metal removed from loosely bound reservoirs Direct removal from metal tightly bound sites occurs but is minimal, even with very potent chelators. days 0-3; 2) symptoms improve from decreased metal content (days 7-14), and 3) re-equilibration (days 21 - 3 months to1 year). Those time points reflect the dominant action, but all 3 of these occur relatively simultaneously. Note the re-equilibration phase is significantly influenced by the amount of heavy metal, and will become clinically apparent as early as 7 days with a massive body load. The observation of three basic time points for various crucial activities of immune response, including healing, also are found for other processes including responses to various foreign invaders/ antigens.

There are 3 large categories of invaders: 1) nonreplicating, which may still increase in amount due to repeated exposure, which heavy metals fall into; 2) replicating foreign invaders, infective organisms (viral, bacterial, fungal) fall into this category;

and 3) replicating internal invaders, cancers and other malignancies are in this category. Heavy metals represent a nonreplicating foreign invader. There is a complex interplay between all these different categories with each other and with the background human organs/ tissues.

Immune Mediated Inflammatory Disease (IMID) and Heavy Metal Toxicity

Abyssus, Abyssum, Invocat. (One Hell calls forth another).

IMID is the current umbrella term for the huge category of diseases which have a major negative action on the immune system and cause an inflammatory reaction, more fully, an immune cell reaction. IMID includes autoimmune diseases (such as Rheumatoid Arthritis and Crohns) and autoinflammatory disease (such as periodic inflammatory conditions an example is TRAPS-Tumor Necrosis Factor Receptor- Associated Periodic Syndrome; I would include IBS Irritable bowel syndrome in this category) and the third category results from a known cause (the use of Auto- suggests the cause is not known) and therefore in this category is Heavy Metal induced IMID. Chronic infections, Lyme, long haul COVID,and mold are also in this third category of IMID, as mentioned above. IMID induced by heavy metals cause a two-hit mechanism of action: The first hit is dysregulating the immune system, which creates the circumstance for the second hit, which is the intrinsic toxicity of the heavy metal.

Most stable (non radioactive) heavy metal toxicities result in this two-hit immunogenicity and toxicity. A negative (harmful) immunogenicity is also termed reactogenicity. Each heavy metal has its own level of effect on immunogenicity (how much it impacts the immune system) and toxicity (its intrinsic toxicity to cells). Within that context different species (subtypes) of heavy metals have different levels of immunogenicity and toxicity. Species describes what the heavy metal is bound to. As an example, inorganic Mercury is mildly toxic, whereas the sub-subtype of the organic Mercuries, Methyl Mercury, is highly toxic. There is a critical nature to the separate contributions of immunogenicity and toxicity, which to date has not been elucidated for each heavy metal.The combined effect of immunity and toxicity has been called autoimmunity with heavy metals, but since the cause is known, it is better classified as Metal-induced IMID. This will be discussed in an upcoming Chapter.

An individual afflicted by an IMID is at heightened risk for developing other IMIDs. Hence Abyssus Abyssum Invocat. This is because IMIDs have the effect of disrupting the normal functioning and responses of the Immune System, termed Immune System Dysregulation (ISD). This dysregulation means that the Immune System may behave in abnormal ways compared to the normal for essentially all immune responses to all entities, such as the response to vaccine injection.

I will illustrate this concept using Gadolinium as the example. Having Gadolinium Deposition Disease (GDD) puts an individual at greater risk for developing other IMIDs. The corollary is also true, having other IMIDs puts one at greater risk for developing GDD. The interconnection between IMIDs and ISD can be visualized as follows: ISD is like a boiling and bubbling internal nebula in the body that has been caused by the presence of IMIDs. Large-content of IMID material, more different IMIDs, and the individual's severity of reaction to these these IMIDs, render the overall picture of ISD more difficult to manage. MRI with Gadolinium Based Contrast Agents (GBCAs) is often used to investigate what is wrong with people with various symptoms and diseases. A large number of the maladies in individuals reflect the presence of other IMIDs and ISD. Therefore GDD is often the last IMID entry into the picture of ISD. As the last entry, GDD is often the most dominant and debilitating.

For the health care provider, it is worthwhile to attempt to determine whether various IMIDs are the entry point to ISD, are bystanders, or are consequence/ exit point of ISD. Staying with the Gadolinium picture, if GDD is the entry point to the creation of ISD, and is relatively mild, then cure with chelation therapy is relatively rapid and complete. If GDD is a later consequence of a combination of varied and severe IMIDs creating ISD, then treatment is more challenging and will require additional ancillary therapies, and significant cure is far less guaranteed.

The clinical plan should center on managing ISD, both its causes and effects, and should be considered in all cases of Heavy Metal Toxicities. Unravelling these various IMID entities carries the prospect of better and more complete treatment. GDD, the toxic state, is almost never a bystander, With Gadolinium and likely all other Heavy Metal Toxicities, the majority of sufferers have at least simple combinations, such as mold toxicity, multiple chemical sensitivity syndrome (MCSS) and Mast Cell Activation Syndrome (MCAS). Some of these, such as mold and MCSS may be entry points to ISD; while others, such as MCAS, may be exit points or consequences of ISD.

Being a bystander means that the entity is present but is not contributing to sickness.The presence of Lyme antibodies is common in GDD sufferers for example, even those unaware that they have ever been infected with Lyme.This may therefore often be a bystander. Lyme antibody presence generally signifies that the body has incorporated Lyme antigens, and the immune system has corralled it, and the infection may or may not have been clinically manifest previously. This is likely the case with a number of additional infective agents. In addition to Lyme, COVID is a common example.COVID may be a bystander, but when the individual has long Haul COVID then it is a common entry point to ISD.

GDD development often opens the Pandora's box of multiple other IMIDs. Another common immunological event is that once a heavy metal IMID has developed, then immune reactions to other metals are activated, such as nickel. This new reaction to other metals, may occur both with newly encountered metals, and also with other heavy metals already present in the body. Previously they may have been quiescent, but now a reaction to them has been activated. There becomes a complex interplay between various IMIDs, and also all these IMIDs and the various organ systems.

Heavy Metals as the cause for chronic inflammatory diseases of unknown etiology:

There are a number of diseases that are considered to have unknown etiology, but in their descriptions, heavy metals are reported as one of the possible causative agents.The most common and/or commonly described are fibromyalgia and ALS, In my opinion a number of these cases represent metal-induced disease. The metal may also be knowable, based on urine studies and response to chelation. A certain percentage of fibromyalgia cases are actually Lead-induced fibromyalgia or Gadolinium-induced fibromyalgia. Similarly certain cases of ALS are actually Lead-induced ALS or Gadolinium-induced ALS. This applies to all the modern descriptions of inflammatory conditions, like Chronic Inflammatory Syndrome or Cytokine Release Syndrome, and multiple others including Stiff Person Syndrome. The critical importance of identifying a heavy metal as the cause for these conditions is that these diseases may then be effectively cured with chelation, as opposed to just lifelong management with anti-inflammatory drugs. In my expert opinion, everyone with these types of disease should undergo a DTPA chelation challenge, looking for the response of a heavy metal removal with associated Flare reactions, and documentation with 24 hour urines pre- and immediately post-chelation.

Further Reading:

1. Bjorklund G, Buha Dordevic A, Hamdan H, Wallace DR, Peana M. Metal-Induced Autoimmunity in Neurological Disorders: A View of Current Understanding and Future Directions. Autoimmunity Reviews 2024; 23: article 103509.

2. Johnson TA, Nguyen LP. .Autoimmunity-Induced Neurotoxicity from Heavy Metals. J Autoimmunity Research 2025; 34: 102-115.

3. Honing DY, Luitin RM, Matos, TR. Regulatory Tcell Dysfunction in Autoimmune Diseases. International Journal of Molecular Sciences 2024; 25: 7171-7185.

4. Schett G, McInnes IB, Neurath MF, et al. Reframing Immune-Mediated Inflammatory Diseases. New England Journal of Medicine 2021; 385: 1302-1314.

CHAPTER

Six

AVOIDANCE.

Chapter 6 Avoidance.
Avoidance.

Avoidance is the basic initial approach for managing toxins including heavy metals. This is a basic element of preventative care. The following are representative examples:

1. Principle strategy for all infectious epidemics of humans throughout the millennia. Avoid close contact with other people. This applies also to vectors for infection: rats, bats, ticks, etc.

In our present age this has been perhaps the most effective tool to deal with COVID: avoid close contact with other people in closed spaces. Extremely few people became ill from COVID in events held in large open spaces. An example was the large open biker rally in South Dakota in 2021. In contrast, over a similar time period, a number of people died from attending closed arena political rallies.

2. Avoid foods, drugs that make you sick/ are allergic too. This is the consistent warning on tv ads for all the expensive Disease-Modifying Anti-Rheumatic Drugs (DMARD), examples Humira,

Stelara, Cosentyx, etc. 'if you are allergic to Humira (or any of its ingredients), don't take it'. How do people know they are allergic to a drug? They don't just wake up one morning and say to themselves "I think I am going to be allergic to Humira, even though I have never taken it". The way they know they are allergic is they have taken it and have experienced a significant reaction to it. If you have shown an allergic reaction to an agent, even after just one exposure, don't take it again.

This applies to sufferers of Gadolinium. Deposition Disease (GDD). The principle treatment is: if you have received a GBCA and have shown the symptoms of GDD, that have persisted over a week, then don't ever receive another GBCA again. This simple strategy would avoid 70% of significant cases of GDD, and atleast 90% of the extremely problematic cases of GDD.

3. Start children on a program of eating healthy food and engaging in moderate activity from the age of 3, starting in preschool. This would avoid obesity in the great majority of individuals. Right now obesity is the major cause of disease, also for all types of diseases, in the world. This may be the single most important health care activity that can be done. In the long run this simple strategy would improve human wellbeing and save trillions of dollars annually.

Complete avoidance of most heavy metals is not feasible as they largely arise from pollution related to living in the modern world. As the steward of your own health you have to focus on minimizing exposure to heavy metals.

Collectively, we have to work to minimize the amount of toxins, including heavy metals, present in the environment and present in foods, medical products, and consumer products.. This generally involves coordinated efforts between government, corporations, and public action groups. Unfortunately in recent decades there have been a number of cases of corporations conducting terrible pollutant releases and with a number, covering this up. Several successful legal actions have pushed back against several corporate misconduct that involved a combination of pollution release, run-off, cover-up with resulting human toxicity and disease.

Specific examples of avoidance and minimization related to heavy metals include:

1. Removal of lead from gasoline in the 1970s.
2. Removal of lead from paint in the 1960s.
3. Removal of Arsenic from chicken feed in the 1990s.
4. Phase out of Mercury in medical devices, thermometers and sphygmomanometers in the early 2000s.
5. Reduction of Cadmium in batteries, starting in 1990s.
6. Stricter regulations of industrial emissions of heavy metals like Cadmium and Nickel in the 1990s and 2000s.

Further Reading::

1.Cheng YF, Zhao Yj, Chen C Zhang F. Heavy Metal Toxicity: Mechanism, Health Effects, and Therapeutic Interventions. Med-Comm 2025; 6: 245-258.

2. Warke M, English M, PAdilla C, et al. Comprehensive Review of In Vitro Approaches for Heavy Metal Exposure. Frontiers of Environmental Science & Engineering 2025; 19:567-580.

3. Li M., Hu J., Zhang Z. Heavy Metal Contamination: Sources, Health Impacts, and Mitigation. International Journal of Environmental Research and Public Health. 2024. 21 2351-2365.

4. Zhao F-J, Jiang R-F, Dunham S J, McGrath S P.. A Review on Heavy Metals Contamination in Soil: Effects, Sources, and Remediation Technologies. 2019. Journal of Soil Contamination & Remediation; 19(6), 1-22.

5. Lanphear B. Lead Poisoning. New England Journal of Medicine 2024; 390: 501-513.

CHAPTER

Seven

DETOXIFICATION.

Chapter 7. Detoxification.

Detoxification. Detoxification is the strategy that focuses on the host and host defences. Detoxification is not the principal form of therapy for heavy metal toxicities. It is however a necessary life skill that is beneficial for an overall regimen of combatting heavy metal toxicity.

Detoxification for all heavy metals, requires a holistic approach that involves managing many contributors to maintaining health: reducing stress, physical activity, restoring the microbiome, and healthy diet are all important elements. Detoxification, as a concept, is both broad and nebulous; and is subject to vagary, uncertainty, and charlatanism. Therefore my approach is that detoxification should be undertaken in the broadest sense: detox for everything, and maybe a number of these efforts will be very beneficial, and hopefully only a few ineffective. Consider diet, microbiome, physical activity, and maintaining mental acuity.

Vagaries include the intention of strengthening the immune system with supplements. The problem with actual strengthening of the immune system, is that although the immune system may then become more effective at combatting proliferating diseases (eg: cancer, infection), but then it will also be more reactive to entities that are immune dysregulating. Therefore a strengthened immune system may make Immune Mediated Inflammatory Diseases (IMIDs) worse. This includes heavy metal toxicity and autoimmune disease. A recurring theme throughout this book is understanding that there is always a critical balance. This is what I term the Goldilocks principle: in this case, strengthening the immune system enough to control proliferating diseases, but not too much to exacerbate IMIDs.

Recommendations:

Decrease stress: One of the worst health disruptors is stress. Reducing stress in all aspects of living is crucial. Even what many people do who are keen on maintaining their health, which is stressing over all aspects of a selected dietary approach (orthorexia), most likely results in an overall negative health effect, than maintaining a more relaxed attitude to striving to eat healthy. The best approach is to follow a reasonable effort to eat a healthy diet, and accept that there may be at least mild toxicity in a number of food items. Another example of unnecessary stress over diet, is worrying over what are the best of the anti-oxidants or the best of the microbiome-restorations. My solution; take a number of different products produced by reputable companies. All in small measure. Guiding principles: everything in moderation and the Goldilocks principle.

Diet: This is broadly considered the core treatment and focus for many diseases. This also has a significant role for combatting Heavy Metal Toxicity: eating a healthy diet. I have termed this concept the **Wholesome Diet** composed of, as best as possible: **Healthy Foods Locally Sourced.** The core understanding is minimizing added sugar and chemical additives (ultraprocessed foods), and paying attention to current scientific knowledge of food safety. The emphasis is on consuming a broad range of foods that have in general some level of anti-oxidant and anti-inflammatory properties, but not too much anti-oxidation (the Goldilocks principle). This is a timeless understanding, maybe understood for thousands of years, and certainly all modern qualified nutritionists essentially extol this. The one critical caveat that most overlook is that attention must be paid to foods that now are no longer healthy, because of pollution or additives/ adjuncts. an excellent example is Kale. Foods with good anti-inflammatory properties include: blueberries, blackberries, pineapple, mango, beans, broccoli, grapes, olives, avocadoes, turmeric, fish, lean beef. and chicken.

Restoring the Digestive System Microbiome: The restoration of a healthy digestive microbiome is among the most important dietary modifications that should be done. This is especially critical for those who may have damaged their microbiome significantly through frequent use of antibiotics. This must however be done sensibly and thoughtfully.

Attempting to restore the microbiome by taking one type of probiotic/biotic may restore/ enhance one healthy organism, but will not create a sufficiently diversified population of microbiomes. Creating a regimen of a number of different products would be sensible. Consume a variety of probiotic and biotic products, and as much as possible ones that seem natural and healthy. Probiotic + biotic yogurts, kefirs, fermented cabbage (sauerkraut, kimchi), in combination with bottled supplement probiotics and biotics.

Physical Activity/ Interventions: Complementary Health Approaches (CHAs): meditation, yoga, and exercises like Tai Chi are all very good. Walking in fresh air and sunlight is a great activity, if you can get it. Moderate activity performed regularly is the best approach.

Physical treatments: Alternative health physical treatments such as acupuncture and hypnosis may be helpful.. Meditation is an obvious inclusion, as it fundamentally is at no charge and easy to do. Religious practices/ prayer are a form of meditation and also are useful.

Sauna can be a useful ancillary treatment. Heavy metals are eliminated in sweat, especially apocrine sweat. Conventional sauna may be better for heavy metals. It is critical to be aware if sufferers have lost the ability to sweat due to the heavy metal (for example Gd) toxicity, sauna can be very toxic. It will heat up the body, without the release mechanism of sweating, resulting in Metabolic Acidosis. Hyperbaric Oxygen Therapy (HBOT) may be of value (except for Chromium Toxicity, where it is dangerous). Ozone therapy may also show benefits, but there is not enough experience yet for me to feel comfortable advocating for it

In people with Immune System Dysregulation (ISD) it is critical when trying any therapy of any kind, start in low amounts and gradually increase. Because of the dysregulation, the response to therapies may be unpredictable, and in fact the opposite of what is intended may occur.

These are 10 commandments of health maintenance:

1. **Hygiene and sanitation** may be the most important advances in health preservation in the modern age, commencing around 1850 in modern Europe and North America. Understanding this importance, ancient Romans practiced this from around 200 BC (BCE) - 400 AD (CE) in western Europe. Cultures like the Japanese have practiced perhaps for millenia without interruption, etc. The general concept is that attention to hygiene and sanitation maintains a general low level of infective and waste material

in the environment and the body, so that undesirable-organism overgrowth does not occur. The feared outcome of overgrowth of toxic organisms and substances is a horrible death.

2. **Healthy natural foods** provides the nutrients that your body requires. The body uses its native, intrinsic metabolic pathways to generate all the important chemicals and proteins it needs for good health.
3. **Moderate exercise and maintenance of joint mobility**. I have espoused Tai Chi and yoga...dancing by yourself... but you can do this in a Zen fashion... which is you decide what to do and how to move your arms and legs, it doesn't need to be formal instruction.
4. **Socialization.** Generally this refers to interactions with other humans. This is an important way to maintain cognitive health and stave off dementia. Maybe the most important in addition to diet. If there is no human around to socialize with, a dog is a good substitute, atleast the dog also shows unconditional love.
5. **Pay attention to family health history.** This will guide you to what you actually will need formal western medicine to maintain health. Family history of high blood pressure, cancer and other malignancies. Know what has happened in your genetic past to predict what there is a good chance that you will experience. If you have the inherited genes for breast cancer (BRCA 1 and BRCA2) or colon cancer (example Lynch syndrome, associated with mismatch repair genes MLH1, MSH2, MSH6, and PMS2)earlier and more consistent screening will be needed, compared to individuals in the general public.
6. **Everything in moderation.** Ignoring this issue is why we are in such a terrible state with **overuse of antibiotics**, with the consequences of antibiotic resistant organisms,

weird parasites, and also the destruction of our native intestinal tract flora (microbiome). Our microbiome has developed and protected humans for over 1 million years, and within a few decades we have greatly destroyed it in many people. **Overuse of opiate drugs** is another example. 100s of thousands of lives lost annually in the USA alone .

7. **Stress reduction.** Prayer and meditation are two means of achieving stress reduction.
8. **Stay away from too many people in closed spaces**. This is especially important in pandemics and epidemics. We learned this again with COVID, but this has been the case throughout all human history with various plagues. The most strikingly named the **Black Death** in the middle ages in Europe. The dose received of an infective organism may be the critical determinant between developing immunity (small dose) and death (large dose). This may be the single most important process for managing/surviving pandemics.
9. **Look for disease if there is a reasonable probability you will have that disease.** As example, if you have had exposure to Asbestos,you will need to undergo some form of surveillance with chest CT. This also relates back to point 5: if there is a strong family history for a disease, there is a high likelihood you may get it as well.
10. **Treat the condition if the condition is problematic (death is the ultimate problem) and treatment has a high probability of working.** Insulin for Type 1 Diabetes, and blood pressure drugs for significant hypertension are good examples. I include GDD and effective chelator treatment in this category

Understand that you are the steward of your own health.

Supplements:

Some supplements may be of value to many individuals with Heavy Metal Toxicity. Overall I prefer the strategy of focusing on eating healthy food to obtain the necessary nutrients.

Recommended supplements: Turmeric; Quercitin; chlorella/spirulina; B complex vitamin; Vitamin C are recommended. A binder such as modified citrus pectin, but I prefer whole fruits oranges, peaches, and apricots apples, pears.

Magnesium: Magnesium will be removed in small amounts with Ca-DTPA, and other chelators. Magnesium is vital for many physiological processes in the body, so removal is not ideal. A number of individuals report that they do better if they receive supplemental Magnesium. My preference is that vitamins and nutrients be consumed as food items that are rich in those chemicals. Magnesium-rich foods include nuts and spinach.

Selenium: Selenium is normal trace element in the body. It is a cationic metal so conceivably could be removed with chelation. The recommendation is to include foods that contain selenium: turmeric, basel, black pepper, and the Brazil nut. Black pepper is an easy addition. The Brazil nut is high in Selenium and other valuable nutrients, so eat Brazil nuts at least on occasion.

Medications: Low Dose Naltrexone (LDN) acts as a mild anti-inflammatory,and a number of Heavy Metal Toxicity sufferers report that it is beneficial. Since heavy metals provoke pro-inflammatory cytokine release, there likely would be considerable benefit using an mTOR inhibitor or Disease Modifying Anti-Rheumatic Drug (DMARD) that targets the cytokines largely involved, similarly a JAK inhibitor, should be effective. To define which one of these agents would be beneficial for which heavy metal would require intensive scientific investigation by experts. Suppressing the wrong cytokines may cause more harm than good. At the time of writing this work, a consistently effective immune system modulating drug has not been identified. Rapamycin, an mTOR inhibitor, as a moderate strength immune suppressor may be of value, but a very low dose is recommended to start. This may be a safer strategy than to use high dose steroids to contain symptoms.

The easiest approach is to start simple: pay attention to eating healthy food, walk often, and when you can, get fresh air and sunshine. Overall show wisdom-sense. It turns out this approach works for all that ails you.

Further Readings::

1.Cheng YF, Zhao Yj, Chen C Zhang F. Heavy Metal Toxicity: Mechanism, Health Effects, and Therapeutic Interventions. MedComm 2025; 6: 245-258.

2. Panda C, Kruse R, Williams K, et al. Metabolic Reset Purification Program Improves Antioxidant Balance and Gut Microbiome in Individuals transitioning to a Healthier Diet. Frontiers in Nutrition 2025; 12: article 1621709.

3. Jayedi A, Soltani S, Emadi A, Zargar M-S, Najafi A. Aerobic Exercise and Weight Loss in Adults. JAMA Network Open, 7: e2412345.

CHAPTER

Eight

REMOVAL. CHELATION.

Chapter 8. Removal. Chelation.
The science of chelation. Measurement of removal.

The fact that metals remain intact and are not degraded in the body are traditionally a significant problem, as classical detoxification will not have much impact on them. However as metals are often in a cation (positive charge) state this makes them very amenable to removal with chelation. Unlike other chemical toxins, which are mainly forever chemicals (for example PFAs), heavy metals also are forever chemicals unless they are chelated out of the body.Chelate is from the Greek for claw, which describes the function of a chelator to grab onto another molecule.

Chelation is the principle method to treat metal diseases because metals cannot be broken down in the body. If an individual is sick from the metal, it needs to be removed in order to improve their health. The way to remove them is for another chemical to bind them to facilitate this. That is chelation.

In general the method of elimination of metals that are chelated is through renal elimination, in most cases, and by hepatobiliary elimination, atleast in part, for some chelators. Hepatobiliary elimination is the process where hepatocytes take up the metal complex and excrete it through bile into the duodenum, and eventually as stool. Metals can also be eliminated in small amounts in other bodily fluids, primarily through sweat, especially apocrine gland, but also through tears, saliva, breathing exhalation, nails, hair, and skin exfoliation. Only sweating results in meaningful elimination. The metal may or may not need to be chelated in these ancillary elimination pathways.

Chelators can either form chemical bonds (generally those that are in the blood circulation) or physical bonds, generally those that are orally taken, remain in the digestive tract, and are eliminated through the digestive tract through fecal elimination. Chelation with chemically bound chelators are the most common.

Common chelators and their types of chemical bonds.

Types of chemical bonds

Covalent bonds. This bonding is formed when atoms share electrons. A form of covalent bonding is **coordinate** bonding where only one atom contributes the electrons to be shared. Coordinate bonding is how the agents DMPS and DMSA bind heavy metals.

Ionic bonds. Virtually all metals are cations (positively charged) in chemical bonds. So when ionic bonds are created the metal is a cation. Chelation then reflects cation exchange bonding, where the chelator exchanges the cation it is manufactured with (most often Ca) with the heavy metal, for example Gd or lead. The term transmetallation has been used in MRI for Gadolinium Based contrast Agent (GBCA) reactions for this process. I find the term confusing so prefer the expression cation exchange.

Electrostatic bonding. Electrical charge without electron shift is electrostatic forces. Illustrations of this are the observations that rubbing a balloon against a wool pant the balloon will stick to the pant leg, or the mild shock of wool to finger touch or hair standing on end putting on a wool sweater in dry climate. Electrostatic bonding combined with molecular folding (like a soft taco) creates the form of bonding that HOPO utilizes..

Administration in active or inactive state

Agents are administered in their active or inactive state, where the latter category has to be converted into active state in the body. This is generally by the liver. DTPA and EDTA are injected in the active state and also eliminated in active form. In contrast DMPS and DMSA are injected as inactive drugs and converted into active form in the liver. This is referred to as agents being prodrugs. There are decided advantages to injection in active forms, as this does not rely on the organ (liver) being healthy for the chelator to function, and also minimizes the risk of toxic damage to organs that detoxify, principally the liver.

Agents with lesser chelation effect

There are a number of supplements, food substances, and drugs with lesser effects of chelation. The most notable are vitamin B subtypes (notably niacin) cilantro, oregano, and emeramide. This category could also include oral physical binders such as pectin, pectin-containing foods, and activated charcoal. Diatomaceous earth is also in this category, but is not recommended because it also contains rare earth metals such as Gd. The B vitamin subtype Niacin has shown efficacy with Arsenic removal, as it assists with methylating Arsenic which facilitates excretion. Deferoxamine is a specific agent that binds to iron to facilitate elimination of iron in urine. This is used in Genetic Hemochromatosis.It is also used with Aluminum. Its use for heavy metals is not recommended as stability is low with them, and will then carry the risk of redistribution. This reflects the chelator picking up the metal then immediately re-releasing it. Penicillamine is used to remove copper in Wilson's Disease.

A problem that can arise with the use of lesser effect chelators, such as cilantro, is it can result in substantial heavy metal redistribution which can worsen heavy metal deposition diseases, such as Gd Deposition Disease. Hence I generally do not recommend weak chelators.

Critical features of an effective chemical chelator.

There are two features that are critical for a chelator to be an effective chelator:

1. The **agent must have high log stability constant** (also termed thermodynamic stability) with the heavy metal in question. This is the strength of the bond, also termed affinity. The target value for a very good chelator is 20.

2. There must be **objective documentation that the chelator removes the heavy metal from the body**. For this purpose we use 24 hour urine testing for 20 heavy metals. Pre-chelation urine obtained within 2 days of chelation, and post-chelation obtained immediately after chelation. The timing for the post-chelation start is after the first urination, which should be either during chelation or immediately after chelation. The explanation why the early urine is not collected, is that this urine would have been created prior to the administration of the chelator. Generally this collection starts at 1 hour post-chelation. The advantage of 24 hour urine is that it shows what actually is removed from the body. A 24 hour acquisition period employs a lengthy window of heavy metal movement and elimination.

Blood (often serum) values for heavy metals also can be used, but since they are snapshots in time of the heavy metal, extreme care must be taken to ensure near exact timing for blood sampling, for comparison to be useful. Probably optimal timing is 45-60 minutes post chelation. Without exact standardization, these values can be misinterpreted as to how much metal is present or removed, and hence dangerously meaningless.

The third point is taken as a given, that it has already been established.

3. The agent must have documented safety.

Selected description of effective chelators in use:

DMSA:

Prodrug. Binds heavy metals with coordinate bonds with sulfhydryl groups. Elimination is through the kidneys. Log stability constant with Mercury= 18, Pb= 18, Gd = 12.. DMSA is a good chelator for mercury and lead, but only fair for Gd.

EDTA:

Active drug. Binds heavy metals with ionic bonds by cation exchange. Elimination is through the kidneys. Log stability constant with Mercury= 12-14, Pb= 18, Gd= 17. EDTA is a good chelator with lead, fair with Mercury, and near good Gd.

DTPA:

Active drug. Binds heavy metals with ionic bonds by cation exchange. Elimination is through the kidneys. Log stability constant with Mercury (inorganic) 26 and (organic)10-14, lead =18.6, Gd= 22. So DTPA is very good with Gd, near very good with lead, extremely good with inorganic but fair with organic mercury. DTPA is the best available chelator for Gd and lead.

HOPO:

Active drug. Binds heavy metals with electrostatic forces and folding over the metal. Elimination is through kidneys and partly hepatobiliary. Log stability constant with mercury= 12-14, lead=

18 , Gd = 20-21. So HOPO is good with lead, very good for Gd, and fair with Mercury,

Prussian Blue:

Active drug. Activity is restricted to the gastrointestinal tract, unlike the above described chelators which work systemically (throughout the body). Prussian Blue is a lattice structured molecule that traps certain cationic elements into its molecular structure. Thallium and Cesium possess molecular structures that can conform to this exchange. Cesium-137 is an element of particular interest because of the radioactivity. This chelator works by interrupting the re-circulation cycle of these elements. Thallium and Cesium are eliminated by hepatobiliary excretion, and in the native state a certain amount of these eliminated heavy metals are re-absorbed in the small intestine, creating recirculation. Prussian Blue interrupts this recirculation by binding Thallium and Cesium in the small intestine, and these chelated metals can no longer be re-absorbed and are eliminated in feces. Its ability to remove other metals that have been incorporated through the gut (which are many of the heavy metals) apparently is minimal. Log stability constant is not described.

Basis of Toxicity:

The principle basis of toxicity for most heavy metals is the combination of creating an Immune Mediated Inflammatory DIsease (IMID) which then facilitates the direct toxic effect, so it is a two-hit mechanism The exact process of how this occurs is not fully understood, however research is ongoing. Components include release of cytokines that induce inflammation, and alteration of cell membrane permeability, either increasing or decreasing cellular entry for a number of chemicals. The IMID creates an environment for passive and active toxic activity. Of equal importance are the Immune system protective mechanisms that prevent the manifestation of the toxic effects. This protected state is termed Heavy Metal Storage Condition. In general Storage

Condition is much more common than the toxic, Deposition Disease state.

Patterns of Response to chelation treatment.

There are 3 patterns reflecting chelator action with heavy metals.

1. **Heavy metal removal**. The higher the log stability the higher the removal. This is the desired activity. This occurs immediately, with the highest effect within 1 hour, but continuing in substantial amounts over day 1, and tapering off by day 3. But minimal continued elimination occurs due to re-equilibration (see below).
2. **Heavy metal redistribution**. This is an undesired effect. This reflects the chelator picking up the heavy metal then immediately releasing it. This occurs with chelators with lower stability, with the lower the stability the larger the amount of redistribution. The effect can be observed by the pick-up of metal in skin, then releasing it right away and the heavy metal traveling to the brain.
3. **Heavy metal re-equilibration**. This represents le Chatelier's principle: everything strives to be in equilibrium. This can be a very effective means of reducing total body heavy metal content. The chelation process removes heavy metals primarily from large reservoirs in which the heavy metal is loosely bound. These are soft tissues: skin, muscles, and organs such as brain, liver, kidneys. This creates an imbalanced state. To re-establish equilibrium. heavy metal in more durable reservoirs, such as bone, shift to the soft tissue reservoirs that had been depleted. Re-equilibration starts likely very soon after chelation, but most often becomes clinically apparent 3 weeks post chelation. Note that continued elimination of heavy metal in urine is also elevated during the re-equilibration period.

Triphasic response to chelation

A triphasic symptom response to chelation has been well established in the peer-reviewed literature for Gd. Less experience with Lead and Mercury has nonetheless shown the same effect. Our opinion is that it is likely observed for many heavy metals.

With an effective chelator the following is observed:

Heavy metal removal Flare Days 0-5.

Period where improvement is observed Days 7-21.

Heavy metal re-equilibration Flare, Days 21-90, tailing off but continuing for 1 yr.

With subsequent chelations, Removal Flare decreases in length and severity, and the period of improvement increases and becomes more sustained. Re-equilibration Flare also diminishes, and this is the critical assessment to determine when to stop chelation.

These 3 phases of symptom responses to chelation is essential to have occurred to establish the definitive confirmation that the patient is sick with a Deposition Disease to the heavy metal. Empirically this is logical: if the individual is sick from the heavy metal, remobilizing it should re-ignite/ intensify the clinical symptoms. Usually these are the symptoms the subject already suffers from, but new types of symptoms may be experienced, that are part of the recognized symptom types associated with the heavy metal. The explanation for new symptom development is that the heavy metal had been retained in multiple tissues including those not initially symptomatic. Immune cells align along all sites of retention, symptomatic or not. Removal from symptomatic sites occurs, because immune cells that cause these symptoms are present there in large numbers. But these immune cells are also aligned in sites that have not previously been symptomatic, and removal now from these sites may also cause symptoms. Aligned immune cells recognize the metal movement and react with cytokine release. Our theory is that tissue resident memory T cells are the primarily tissue based immune cells. Each organ system has their own type of resident memory T cells. Removal Flare may be negligible in some sufferers, and re-equilibration Flare more noticeable. The period of improvement may take a number of sessions for definite positive change to be appreciated.

If a subject does not have Deposition Disease then removal of the metal and re-equilibration will not cause symptoms. Presently the presence of these symptoms is the most definitive finding to confirm toxicity/ Deposition Disease. Their absence reflects Storage Condition.

The critical determination of when to pause/ stop chelation is when the re-equilibration Flare is mild at 1 month post chelation and remains mild at 3 months. It is not however rare that a second shorter stretch of chelation sessions may be necessary about 1 year post the last chelation, as the ongoing continuous re-equilibration of bone back to soft tissues may eventually cause a recurrence of symptoms after 9 months. Since the total body content of heavy metal will have been greatly diminished from the earlier chelation sessions, only few further chelations are necessary, usually 3 suffices. Through the periods of re-equilibration it should also be noted that there is also increased native elimination of heavy metal, since heavy metal must pass through the circulation to move from bone to soft tissues, and a fair amount of this moving metal in circulation will also be removed by the kidneys.

Noteworthy is that a triphasic response is very common for a variety of physiological events in the body. The best example is the healing for skin wounds, and other wounds. In these cases, the 3 components do the following: i) tissue destruction, ii) massive fibrin production, iii) remodeling. As with removal and re-equilibration, with skin healing these 3 processes occur at the same time, but the relative proportion of these actions varies with time, like a ballet performance. Re-equilibration of heavy metals likely begins within 24 hours of removal, but it does not become clinically apparent in most individuals till 3 weeks. In the case of massive heavy metal deposition the clinical manifestation can appear sooner, such as at 1 week. This is because re-equilibration Flare arises on the basis of how much of the heavy metal is present, and therefore in motion with chelation, to elicit the intense inflammatory response of re-equilibration Flare.

Immunological effects as separate from toxic

An important aspect of Heavy Metal Toxicity is that it represents a combined immunologic/toxic effect, which is a two-hit mechanism. For heavy metal toxicity to occur there is always a two-hit process. While the dose of the heavy metal is extremely important to develop toxicity/ Deposition Disease (Paracelsus- the dose makes the poison), the immunology response to the metal is the important initiating effect. Heavy metal in a contained space, even a small amount, can cause Deposition Disease. Using Gd in GBCAs as an illustration, contained extravasation of a GBCA in soft tissues of the arm, or the localized Gd in an MR arthrogram, the latter often containing no more than 1 ml of GBCA, can cause the disease. How this happens is due to the immunological response. The exact analogy is a vaccination against viruses. The vaccine is administered in a small dose but in a contained location such as intramuscular, subcutaneous, intradermal, where sufficient numbers of antigen-presenting (eg: dendritic) cells can congregate at the site and pick up sufficient numbers of the antigen to take back to lymph nodes and show to enough T cells to create an immune response. Vaccine administered in the blood stream through a vein would disperse too extensively for enough antigen-presenting cells to pick them up. This explains why vaccines are not injected intravenously. This also accounts exactly for the immunologic effect of a heavy metal.

Laboratory confirmation.

24 hour urine documentation of heavy metal content pre- and post-chelation are an objective demonstration of the effect of a chelator, and is essentially as scientific documentation of effect as any test in medicine. It is noteworthy that post-chelation urine content remains high for the heavy metal until the largest durable reservoir has been depleted. This is clearly shown for Gd. This also represents a useful documentation of decreasing the total body reservoir of other heavy metals. This is the important clinical result. Using Gd as the example, when post chelation urine has decreased from upwards of 20 mcg/ 24 hours to 3 mcg/ 24 hour this is supportive evidence that bone content of Gd, and by extension total body Gd content, is now significantly depleted. Re-equilibration can no longer deliver enough Gd from bone back to soft tissues to maintain high post-chelation numbers, because the Gd content in bone has been greatly diminished. The Gd content in post-chelation 24 hr urine remains stable at high levels for multiple chelation sessions, because of the effective restoration of Gd content to soft tissues by re-equilibration from the large bone repository. Decrease of 24 hour post-chelation urine Gd stays moderately high until the bone reservoir is significantly depleted. Often this occurs after 5 chelation sessions, but in the case that the individual has a lot of Gd in their body, from 10 or more GBCA injections, the persistent high amount of Gd post-chelation in the urine may remain for upwards of 10- 15 chelations.

X-ray fluorescence spectroscopy (SR-XRF) can demonstrate Gd and other metals in cortical bone. This has to date been restricted to bone that is very superficial to skin, because of limited penetration of these x-rays. Tibia has been examined most often for this technique.

Prior research studies looking at cytokine release in subjects who have received GBCA injection, have shown elevation of cytokines post chelation. Perhaps the most interesting are the dynamic serial acquisition of cytokines, which at present have been only performed by our team to look at Gd, At present an insufficient number of patients have been studied to determine definitive findings. The current theory is that the total amount of cytokine release reflects the total amount of Gd remobilized from the tissues, which is based on how much Gd is present in the body. This generally reflects the number of GBCA injections. This total amount of cytokines does not distinguish Storage Condition (not sick) from Deposition Disease (sick) More clear definition of the types of cytokines that distinguish disease from storage states has yet to be established. Intuitively a greater amount of pro-inflammatory cytokines are released in patients with disease, and more inflammation suppressing cytokines in subjects with storage condition.

Radioactivity

A number of the heaviest heavy metals also are radioactive, for example Plutonium. The principal concern with these metals is not the immune mediated inflammatory disease (IMID) - toxic combined effect that most stable heavy metals cause, but the deterministic (meaning consistent for everyone) damaging effect of radiotoxicity. Radiotoxicity is more rapid and lethal, and generally all individuals exposed to a radioactive metal experience this injury, rather than the estimated 1 in 10,000 who experience IMID/toxicity from nonradioactive stable metals. Safety and concern for removing native metals are crucial considerations when chelating stable metals such as Gd and lead, hence the chelation regimen is a slow process with relatively long gaps. In contrast, rapid removal of radioactive metals is necessary to limit the destructive process of radiation. Zn-DTPA is currently considered for removal of Plutonium, because daily chelation can be performed with minimal removal of native metals. I would recommend the use of Ca-DTPA because it removes more heavy metal than Zn-DTPA, approximately twice as much, and this likely is very important to minimize the destruction that the radiation will cause. Daily Ca-DTPA will remove some native metals, so a regimen that incorporates replenishment of native metals is essential. An approach like 3 days Ca-DTPA then 1 day native metal restoration, and multiple repetitions of this regimen .

Chelation Protocols

There are two fundamental principles that form the basis of generating protocols for chelation:

1. **Total body heavy metal burden**. Where are the major reservoirs of the metal retention in the body? How durable are these reservoirs, which is to say how tightly bound is the heavy metal in specific reservoirs and therefore how difficult to remove.

2. **Le Chatelier's Principle.** Everything strives to be in equilibrium. Removal of heavy metals from durable reservoirs is more difficult, and often must rely on le Chatelier's principle to shift the heavy metal to more removable sites. The rate this re-equilibration occurs will also determine the intervals between chelation sessions. Because of this step-wise process of removing total body content of heavy metal, multiple chelation sessions is always required in sufferers. Generally 5 sessions is the minimum for most (all) heavy metals.

These concepts are well established for the bone-reservior dominant heavy metals lead and Gd, and also apply to Cadmium, which is also a bone-reservoir dominant heavy metal.. Likely these are similar for other heavy metals, but not established. This will be discussed in chapters on the metals themselves.

Route and rate of exposure to the heavy metal,

The use of DTPA perhaps best illustrates these points. DTPA is FDA-approved for the removal of Plutonium, Americium, and Curium, all radioactive heavy metals. Some of the earliest use of DTPA was for accidents in radiation plants, and the notable exposure was inhalation of Plutonium. Treating doctors at that time employed an empirically logical delivery of chelator by aerosolized inhalation of DTPA. In settings where radioactive metals are inhaled, they will also have experienced cutaneous exposure. So aerosolized chelation treatment could be supplemented with cutaneous (skin) application.

The current widespread use of DTPA is for off-label chelation of Gd and lead. The method of exposure for the vast majority of cases of Gd exposure is near unique among heavy metals. The exposure is for medical reasons, by intravenous administration of a bound (chelated) form of Gd. Another critical aspect is that the GBCAs are administered as a fast injection, generally 2 ml/sec, and not by a slow drip rate. The reason for the fast injection is that it drives the Gd into the deep extracellular matrix ((ECM) also called interstitial space) so that well vascularized cancers, and other processes such as inflammation become more obvious due to intense enhancement (brightening) on a type of MR sequence (T1 sequences). Drip infusion, tried in the earliest days of GBCA use (early 1990s), does not reveal that clear distinction of brighter appearance of cancers compared to background organs. This brighter appearance not only allows more confident diagnosis, but at times the only way to see these diseases. Fast administration of GBCA is unquestionably important. Administration therefore of DTPA should follow not only the route (intravenous) but also the rate (fast bolus) as the GBCA had entered the body. There are roles for slower drip infusion of chelator, such as extreme sensitivity to Gd, the subject does not want to receive steroids to manage Flare, and later in a series of chelations, in which a fair amount of the Gd is now from re-equilibration (which a higher proportion is vessel wall based, as re-equilibration is at the slower rate of bloood flow) and not just from the original administration.

Most other heavy metals have been incorporated into the body by oral digestive tract exposure, example lead. Inhalation and skin contact are less frequent routes, and generally observed in nuclear accidents. DTPA is presently only available as an iv administration, since there is no oral form of DTPA manufactured as yet. Although intravenous administration of an active agent ensures 100% bioavailability; the benefit of intravenous administration is not as essential for the treatment of orally acquired or inhalational/cutaneous acquired heavy metals.

Mud Tracks.

Mud trucks is a pictorial description of the above considerations of route and rate of administration. This reflects how the heavy metal exposure occurred and hence the pathway that heavy metal is deposited along in the body. The mud tracks follow the path of administration.

To illustrate this issue: Gd given by intravenous administration develops mud tracks of Gd along all vessels arteries, capillaries, veins throughout the entire course of the vascular system. The densest concentration (thickest mud tracks) along capillaries and small veins (venules), because these locations experienced more prolonged contact and transfer of Gd between vessel and tissue and vice versa. The fast injection drives GBCAs into the ECM, so mud tracks are also present in the ECM. The mud tracks of lead would follow how it was incorporated, so mud tracks along the digestive tract, most along small bowel, then the vessels that transport blood from the small bowel, which are small branches of superior mesenteric vein, to portal vein, to liver, so the thickest mud tracks would follow that distribution.

Bioavailability

This property describes how much of the agent that is administered, in this case the chelator, is actually absorbed into the body, Bioavailability is a key measure with orally administered drugs. The relationship of the amount delivered and the amount incorporated is generally expressed as a percentage. So of the 100% of a drug taken orally, the percentage that is actually incorporated. Ideal would be >80%, very good around 50%. If the bioavailability is very low, such as 5%, this can be compensated for by taking more of the agent, if this is safe. The same analysis would be made for cutaneous, lung, rectal drug administrations. Aerosolized lung administration of an agent generally would achieve much higher bioavailability, since the lung parenchyma has thin tissue separating lung from vessels.

Prodrugs, are agents that need to be converted into active form in the body. This represents an additional variable of bioavailability, because the agent needs to be activated in the body. The health of the drug-converting organ affects the extent and rate of conversion. Both DMSA and DMPS are converted into active form by the liver, hence a diseased liver (acute or chronic hepatitis, cirrhosis) would be much less capable of making the activating conversion, hence much lower bioavailability. The additional problem is a drug that is transformed in a diseased liver, carries a significant risk of making the liver disease worse.

Multimetal Toxicity/ Deposition Disease

The clear advantage of intravenous DTPA over other chelators is that it has higher stability with more heavy metals. So at the present time even though DTPA is administered by iv, and most metals other than Gd, are orally acquired, DTPA is still the chelator of choice. This is because DTPA has much higher stability of the combination of Gd (stability=21), lead (17.6) and Cadmium (19), than other available chelators.

Future

This review of chelators provides state of the art knowledge of heavy metals where chelation science is clearly shown, notably Gd, and describing where scientific improvements are necessary. Purpose-made chelators need to be created for specific metals, in which existing broad-spectrum chelators may not be sufficiently effective. Mercury, Arsenic, Chromium, and Platinum are examples. Combination of chelators may be necessary in some settings of multi-heavy metal deposition disease. Efforts to develop laboratory tests (eg:lymphocyte proliferation test) and to identify patterns of cytokine release to distinguish accurately Deposition Disease from Storage Condition are critical.

Further Reading:

1.Semelka RC, Ramalho M. Gadolinium Toxicity and Current State of Knowledge and Expert Opinion. Investigative Radiology 2023; 58: 233-245

2.Cheng YF, Zhao Yj, Chen C Zhang F. Heavy Metal Toxicity: Mechanism, Health Effects, and Therapeutic Interventions. Med-Comm 2025; 6: 245-258.

3. Domingo JL, Semelka RC. Gadolinium Toxicity:Mechanisms, Clinical Manifestations, and Nanoparticle Role. Archives of Toxicology 2025; 99: 3897-3916.

4. Martell AE, Smith RJ. authors.Title: Critical stability constants, Vol 6: Second Supplement. Plenum Press, NY, NY. 1992.

CHAPTER

Nine

TISSUE/ORGAN LOCATIONS OF RETENTION

Chapter 9. Tissue/organ locations of principle retention (deposition). Durability of metal retention in various organs/ tissues. Transient vs Persistent Metal Presence. Total body heavy metal content and removal.

Localization of retention:

Exact locations of heavy metals throughout organs and tissues throughout the human body is at present unknown, but reasonable estimates for some of these heavy metals have been derived, using a combination of animal studies, regional tissue studies in humans, and cadaver studies in humans. Perhaps the best established is the findings for Gd. Approximately 40% in bone, 35% in skin, 15% in muscle, 5% in brain, 5% in primarily liver and kidneys, and minimal in lungs.

The literature on Lead suggests 95% is retained in bone. My opinion is that this estimate is incorrect, and numbers are more closely aligned to Gd, where for Lead, 65% is in bone, 10% in skin,

10% in muscle, and 15% primarily in brain, liver, kidneys, and minimal in lungs.

Cadmium probably follows Lead quite closely.

Mercury tends to store in kidneys, brain, and fatty tissue .

Beryllium is generally incorporated through inhalation, so 90% would be retained in the lungs, and 10% in other soft tissue organs, notably the kidneys.

Durability of retention:

The durability of retention in various organs largely depends on how impacted the metal is into the organ. Bone having a crystalline matrix, heavy metals such as Gd, {ead, and Cadmium can be both trapped in that matrix, but also can insert themselves into that matrix by substituting for Calcium.

In general, the larger the percentage of heavy metal in a durable matrix, the more chelation sessions are required to achieve adequate clinical improvement, and the greater the reliance on le Chatelier's principle to reduce total body heavy metal removal.

Transience vs Persistence of heavy metal presence:

The property of how long metals stay in the body, transience vs persistence, is an important concept. Transient metals generally do not require any particular treatment. The requirement of treatment depends both on the durability and toxicity of metals. Toxicity for a particular metal can vary dramatically between individuals.

Bismuth is an excellent example of a transient metal. Taken orally (for example Pepto Bismol) in the short term there can be a significant elevation in the urine,which means it has been incorporated into the vascular system, yet it decreases rapidly to 0 within a couple of days.

Transience of heavy metals is well documented with serial urine studies. For example, comparing pre-chelation 24 hour urine within 2 days of DTPA chelation with post-chelation urine, which are performed to evaluate for Gd and lead removal, allows for assessment of how effective the chelator has been to remove metals.These same urine studies can be used to assess transience. As an example. Pepto Bismol taken 1 day prior to pre-chelation urine testing, shows a peak of urine Bismuth at that time point which can be high, but 3 days later on the post-chelation urine, the amount of Bismuth is low. This pairing of urine results is effective at revealing that the metal presence was transient. Metals that are spontaneously eliminated, but not aided by chelation with DTPA, observing on native (unprovoked) urine studies, steady presence of a heavy metal shows that it has persistence. This can be seen with Uranium and Platinum as examples. A low level on prechelation (native) urine does not mean that the body content of the metal is low. This may mean that the heavy metal is bound in tissues and is not leaking out on its own. This same interpretation can be made with post-chelation urine values, a low level post chelation may mean that the chelator is not effective at removing the heavy metal, and the total body content may actually be quite high.

Classical durable metals have bone as a major repository, and these are Gd, Lead, and Cadmium.

Total body heavy metal content

Total body heavy metal content is a critical concept for all metals. Unfortunately there is little direct evidence in living humans how much heavy metal is present, retained within tissues, or how much is present in various organs and tissues. Therefore surrogate evidence must be used. A finding that provides useful information after an acute exposure is 24 hour native (unprovoked) urine measurement. Blood levels are also of value in this setting. On 24 hr native urine testing in a steady state (no recent intense exposure to a heavy metal) the amount of heavy metal shown is not a reflection of how much is present in the body, but rather how much is being decorporated (leaving the body) on its own. On postchelation 24 hour urine measurements, the amount shown provides evidence of presence, and of effectiveness of the chelator to remove that metal, but not of the total body burden as such. However, a very high number, > 200 mcg/24 hr, is indicative that an enormous amount of Gd is present.

To illustrate the subject of presence and removal with chelation, Thallium has a stability constant of 10 with DTPA, which reflects that DTPA is a relatively poor chelator for this metal. If Thallium does not show much increased elimination from prechelation urine to post, this does not mean that there is no significant body burden of Thallium, this reflects that DTPA is a poor chelator for this metal. It should be noted that Thallium does show good native elimination in urine (and stool), reflecting that it is not stored in durable reservoirs, such as bone. Strength of a chelator for heavy metal removal on the other end of the spectrum, is shown by DTPA use for Gd removal. DTPA has high affinity for Gd so the extent of Gd removal and the level of Gd content on 24 hr post-chelation urine study gives an appreciation of how much Gd is present in an individual. The exception is the most stable GBCAs (see chapter on Gd). In contrast, the use of a weaker chelator, such as DMSA, may show Gd remaining low on post-contrast 24 hr urine. This does not mean there is no substantial amount of Gd present, it may simply reflect that a poor chelator was used.

Therefore the surrogate I use for determining total body Gd and Lead content, but more correctly when the total body content has significantly depleted with chelation, is to observe when post-chelation 24 hr urine content drops significantly into the low intermediate range of Gd and Lead content. This reflects that the bone Gd and Lead content, the largest and most durable reservoir, has been significantly depleted such that it can no longer restore a substantial amount of Gd and Lead back to soft tissues.

A typical pattern of 24 hr urine measurements for Gd, for the linear GBCAs and Gadavist look something like this: stable at 25 mcg for 5 chelations sessions, dropping to 17 mcg for 2 sessions, dropping to 10 mcg for 2 sessions, dropping to 5 mcg, then dropping to 3 mcg. For these measurements to be comparable between studies, it is important to pay attention to the chelation intervals, The most accurate comparison is when chelation sessions are spaced constant, at 3 or 4 weeks for example. This is in order to use change in urine Gd content as a standardized marker. The amount of Gd in urine postchelation not only reflects the amount of Gd in the body, but also reflects the interval between chelations. The shorter the interval, the less time has been allowed for Gd to re-equilibrate from bone back to tissues. Therefore post chelation urine values will be lower. The opposite effect is observed with longer intervals. The longer the interval the more re-equilibration has occurred, and hence the higher the amount of Gd in the postcontrast urine. This is worth emphasizing: postchelation urine Gd, Lead and Cadmium drop dramatically when the bone content, the largest and most durable reservoir for these metals, starts dropping significantly. This reflects that the bone reservoir no longer has sufficient Gd, Lead or Cadmium to restore the soft tissue reservoir after chelation, by le Chatelier's principle. This then is a reliable marker that the total body content of these metals has greatly reduced.

Further Reading:

1. Lanphear B. Lead Poisoning. New England Journal of Medicine 2024; 390: 501-513.

2.Semelka RC, Ramalho M. Gadolinium Toxicity and Current State of Knowledge and Expert Opinion. Investigative Radiology 2023; 58: 233-245.

3. Murata N, Murata K, Gonzalez-Cuyar LF, et al. Gadolinium Tissue Deposition in Brain and Bone. Investigative Radiology 2016; 51: 671-678.

4.Cheng YF, Zhao Yj, Chen C Zhang F. Heavy Metal Toxicity: Mechanism, Health Effects, and Therapeutic Interventions. MedComm 2025; 6: 245-258.

5. Domingo JL, Semelka RC. Gadolinium Toxicity:Mechanisms, Clinical Manifestations, and Nanoparticle Role. Archives of Toxicology 2025; 99: 3897-3916.

CHAPTER

Ten

HOW TO TREAT. WHEN TO TREAT. WHEN TO STOP.

Chapter 10- How to treat. When to treat. When to stop. Multimetal Treatment. Radioactive Metal Treatment.

There have not been established criteria on chelation: how to treat, when to chelate, and when to stop. The impression I have is that most practices chelate because heavy metal is present in urine, use chelators that they can readily purchase, and stop chelating when the patient no longer returns. There are however objective criteria for these decisions, and this will be discussed in this chapter. This chapter describes criteria for how to treat, when to chelate, and when to stop.

How to Treat

Heavy metals have particular nuances on how to treat them. These are several of the important factors:

1) the chelator used must have high affinity for the metal(s) of interest. The log stability constant between chelator and metal must be known by the chelation center, and the chelator with the highest log stability constant used. A good target number is 20.

2) there must be documentation that the chelator is actually removing the metal in the individual.We use 24 hr urine pre- and post-chelation.

3) appropriate intervals must be used between chelations, which includes allowing time for the body and native metals to recuperate and paying attention to Le Chatelier's principle and the re-equilibration timeline of transfer of the metal from the largest durable reservoir back to more loosely bound reservoirs,

4) a certain type of detoxification may have particular benefit for a certain metal.

Appropriately performed chelation serves as the principle therapy for most heavy metals. .

When to treat:

1) **If something is making you sick, remove it**.

2) for certain metals some species are very toxic, others not. If a toxic isotope (subtype of the metal) is present, chelation should be performed. Cesium-137 is radioactive and should be treated. Stable Cesium generally does not need to be treated, and simply avoiding foods like kale is often sufficient..

3) the first chelation session is the indicator that treatment is necessary. If chelation with an effective chelator results in Removal Flare and Re-equilibration Flare, chelation is necessary because the patient is toxic from the metal.

4) In general, if native (unprovoked) urine value is in the red range of content in 24 hour study, beyond 1 month of exposure, chelation should be considered.

Urine Testing for Documentation: This provides scientifically valid data. This is effectively done by 24 hour heavy metal testing, in a very short time before chelation, I use within 3 days. Postchelation 24 hour urine starts after the first urination following chelation. The first urination may be during the iv chelation, and hopefully shortly after completion of iv chelation Collection should aim to start 1 hour after chelation completion. This same start time should be used for oral chelators.We start after the first urination, because that urine will primarily contain urine created before the chelator was administered. This concept is obvious and straightforward: keep timing accurate and consistent for comparison purposes.

Regarding urine measures, we always use 24 hrs. The reasons include that there is likely a circadian (variation over 24 hours) pattern of native heavy metal elimination in urine. Since that pattern has not been established, to avoid introducing an additional variable of uncertainty, the simplest approach is to collect the entire 24 hours. So a test fraught with a number of variables (basically every test is) to remove an important variable is wise. On 24 hour measurements labs report heavy metal content in mcg/ g Cr as well as mcg/ 24 hours. I prefer the measure mcg/24 hours because that is clear to understand.Collection times less than 24 hr generally only report heavy metal content in mcg/ g Cr, and not mcg/ time point, which is another reason I do not like lesser time collections than 24 hours. It is not clear what mcg/ g Cr means, because the content of urine Cr is also subject to variables. So who knows what mcg/ gCr means, but a total amount removed in 24 hrs is clear. Interestingly though the relative increases in measures of heavy metals on charts of mcg/ g Cr looks nearly identical to charts of mcg/ 24 hrs, even though labs claim that mcg/ g Cr cannot be converted to mcg/ 24 hr. Whatever the case, I prefer actual quantities, and I like taking out the circadian pattern from a test which already has a number of uncontrolled variables. So that explains 24 hr urine collection.

Blood testing, not preferred: Serum levels for heavy metals are often used by many centers. I do not utilize them, and for the following reasons: cost; convenience (the sufferer may have to go to an offsite lab); the amount of Gd in a blood sample is far lower than in a 24 hour urine sample, so a low but real blood content will not be detected; pain from needle poke; concern of thrombosis of veins, since for many heavy metals vessel deposition is common and heavy metal deposition in venous walls both causes heightened pain sensitivity and also higher likelihood of thrombosis; blood sampling represents a snapshot in time; regarding a snapshot, the best timing for the snapshot is not known; it is absolutely critical to obtain the most reliable and best time shot between studies; exact timing of blood acquisition is critical and must be consistent between chelation sessions; blood sampling reveals the presence of the heavy metal in blood, but not the amount coming out of the body, and the amount coming out is what is important with chelation. So numerous points why I don't favor serum measures. That said, the time point post chelation I would use for blood sampling is exactly 45-60 minute window post each tested chelation.

A science-based documentation of the lower sensitivity of blood sample than 24 hr urine to detect Gd has been reported by a few researchers with Gd. Following 1 GBCA injection blood value for Gd is undetected by 2 months, whereas Gd detection in urine in the same individuals will be continued to be observed in 24 hr urine for at least 3 months.

Amount of Chelator

The safe amount of chelator that can be used has not been determined. As such, I do not advise testing the limits of safety.

A preliminary report on the use of DTPA as a chelator found that weekly intervals of a two day chelation session involving one vial (5 ml/ 1 g) Ca-DTPA day 1; and one vial (5 ml/ 1 g) Zn-DTPA day 2 showed that at 1 week post chelation the values of electrolytes were normal. This would be the shortest interval we would use. One week intervals probably are safest if just Zn-DTPA is used as a 1 day chelation. To maximize safety, and also bone Gd and Lead removal we employ 3-4 week intervals between chelations. With 9 years of clinical experience this two-day regimen has been tolerable for the great majority of patients. Attention has to be paid to how sensitive an individual is to Gd, Lead, Cadmium, Mercury,which is shown by how intense the removal and re-equilibration Flares are. This explains why our present practice is to start with a low dose of chelator (typical 1/2 vial Zn-DTPA) and full regimen of steroids/antihistamines. We then increase chelator from there, and decrease steroids for subsequent chelations.

The end goal for most patients is full dose Ca-DTPA day 1, full dose Zn-DTPA day 2. Smaller size individuals may not tolerate this amount of chelators, and half doses may be necessary.

Similar attention to regimens using other chelators, such as DMSA, should be employed. We describe these regimens in chapters on heavy metals where DMSA or other chelators are advised.

Intervals between chelation sessions:

For heavy metals in which bone is the dominant durable reservoir of metal, this includes: Gd, Lead, and Cadmium, optimal timing takes two properties into consideration: 1) enough time for the body to re-establish homeostasis (all electrolytes returned to a normal level), a safe lower limit for this is 1 week, and 2) enough time for re-equilibration to occur such that sufficient heavy metal has moved from bone back to soft tissues. This re-equilibration is critical, since chelators are most efficient at removing heavy metals from soft tissues, and there is little direct removal from bone. In general 3-4 weeks is optimal timing for most sufferers, since enough time has passed to allow a fair amount of heavy metal to move from bone back to soft tissues, that then can be removed with the upcoming chelation, and not too much time has elapsed that uncontrolled re-equilibration Flare has occurred. It has been through the observation that re-equilibration Flare starts at about 21 days in most people, that this re-equilibration timeline of chelation intervals has been determined. Chelation removal of total body content of Gd, Lead, and Cadmium follows this stepwise reduction of heavy metal.

One nuance is that individuals with a large Gd load, and this would be the case for Lead and Cadmium, substantial re-equilibration is achieved much earlier. This is because there is simply so much heavy metal present, that a large amount is removed by chelation and then a subsequent large amount is re-equilibrated from bone to re-establish equilibrium. The large re-equilibrating amount therefore is symptomatically appreciated earlier on, since already a large amount of Gd would have been mobilized. Individuals with > 15 GBCA injections, re-equilibration Flare may be very apparent at 10-14 days. In those cases intervals between chelation should decrease so chelations are spaced to when re-equilibration becomes very noticeable (10-14 day intervals for example).

Very short intervals, such as daily, I generally do not favor. For example if Zn-DTPA is used to chelate individuals who have received a weaker bond linear agent, such as Omniscan or Magnevist, since this agent is sufficiently effective to remove these agents, a significant amount of Zn is left behind. Although one dose of substantial Zn left behind resolves at one week's time, it is unclear to me how effective native homeostasis can manage piling on of more excess Zn. The physiological impact is uncertain. This will be elaborated further in the chapter on Gd.

If Ca-DTPA is used daily, then clinically evident removal of native metals like Manganese (Mn), Magnesium (Mg), and Zinc will occur and this may have deleterious effects. 3 week intervals allow sufficient time for homeostasis to return these metals to normal values.

The exception to when daily chelation should be used is for radioactive heavy metals. The concern for life threatening radiation damage exceeds the concern of disordering balance of native heavy metals. Since Ca-DTPA removes more Gd (by extrapolation also more Plutonium), approximately twice as much asZn-DTPA. I would employ a regimen that includes stretches of repeat daily Ca-DTPA, interspersed with1 day of native metal restoration - so 3 consecutive days of Ca-DTPA followed by 1 day of electrolyte recovery, with multiple repetitions.

Because of the requirement of re-equilibration to achieve total body heavy metal removal of Gd, Lead, and Cadmium, it is always necessary to perform multiple repeat chelation sessions to accomplish substantial total body removal. For the great majority of individuals this is a minimum of 5 chelation sessions. Generally 5 chelation sessions are required for each GBCA injection, so 5 GBCAs means 25 chelation sessions. These chelation sessions should be spaced 3-4 weeks apart.

Heavy metals for which bone is not the dominant durable repository then this timeline of chelation session intervals would be adjusted, and generally to shorter intervals, since fat for example does not retain heavy metals as tenaciously as bone does. Shorter intervals between chelations can be used.

Ca-DTPA day 1/ Zn-DTPA day 2.

Ca-DTPA removes more heavy metal than Zn-DTPA, but it also removes native heavy metals: Mn, Mg, Zn. Zn-DTPA day 2 then restores Zn removed by Ca-DTPA, does not remove additional native metals, while also continuing the removal of more heavy metal. In my theory this includes heavy metal loosened but not removed day 1. We use the analogy that heavy metals are like stones in a stream bed, the flushing of the stream bed by Ca-DTPA removes a lot of the stones, but loosens others, before these stones can reset, the second flush of Zn-DTPA day 2 captures a number of the loosened stones (heavy metal particles). We typically pulse administration of DTPA as two separate hand-pushed boluses for each of the two chelators. As mentioned elsewhere this method of administration of chelators mirrors how the GBCA was administered in the first place. This approach is important for Gd, it is not clear that it is as important for Lead or Cadmium, since these were incorporated through the digestive tract, and hence were not forced deep into the extracellular matrix (ECM), which was the case with Gd. Nonetheless bolus injection is still better than drip injection to remove heavy metals from the deep ECM, so probably should be used for most cases.

Steroids/ antihistamines

Individuals who are sick from heavy metals, that is are experiencing toxicity (also described as Deposition Disease) will always also react when an effective chelator is used and the heavy metal is pulled out of its location in soft tissues.My theory is that tissue resident memory T cells react to the removal of Gd (also Lead, Cadmium) from tissues and the ECM. The metals pulled out of tissues then enter the blood circulation which then causes an immune reaction by blood circulating T cells and other immune cells. If an individual is not sick from the heavy metal, there is no impetus for this inflammatory reaction, hence steroids/ antihistamines are not needed. If an individual who is not toxic but wants to have heavy metals removed (Storage Condition state), perhaps because they have a lot of Gd or Lead in them, then this does not need to be accompanied with steroids/ antihistamines, because by definition they do not react with cytokines that are pro-inflammatory.

Heavy metal Re-equilibration Flare, to establish re-equilibration (le Chatelier's principle), arises when re-equilibration from bone back to soft tissues occurs (in earnest around 21-28 days). My theory for the immune reaction is the combination of: 1) movement of heavy metal out of bone, 2) heavy metal transit in circulation, and 3) heavy metal implanting back in soft tissues,

The use of steroids and antihistamines reflects the recognition that the Flares are immune reactions, so use of the standard approach of Acute Hypersensitivity Reactions (AHRs) is appropriate.

Redistribution Flare occurs when a low stability chelator is used for chelation. The chelator releases the metal back into the circulation, so the metal picked up in skin may be redeposited in the brain, as example. This explains why we never recommend a lower stability chelator when a higher stability chelator is available.

Steroids: We employ a combination of iv steroids concurrent with chelation, and oral steroid taper afterwards. As the effects of high dose and long duration steroids can be very deleterious, the plan is to decrease steroids as rapidly and judiciously as possible. So the oral steroid use is given as a decreasing taper.The first step in decreasing the amount of steroid used is to replace the iv steroids with oral steroids during chelation. The next step is to drop the amount and number of days of the postchelation oral steroid taper. Low dose steroids can also be restarted if re-equilibration Flare is severe, such as 4 mg Methylprednisolone from days 21-28 with chelation on day 28..

The steroid we traditionally use is Methylprednisolone, both in iv and oral form. A sizable number of people with metal toxicity, maybe 1/3, also have MTHFR gene variant. This means they have decreased ability to methylate drugs, and the methylation process in the body is a common mechanism to make the drug (in this case steroid) effective. Administering drugs already in the methylated state makes these agents more effective in MTFHR individuals. Giving everyone methylated drugs also takes knowing whether or not a person has the MTHFR gene variant, out of the equation. Everyone is treated as if they may have this, with no downside for anyone.

Antihistamines. In simple GDD without significant other Immune Mediated Inflammatory Diseases (IMIDs) and a mild severity of Immune System Dysregulation (ISD) the impact of antihistamines is not substantial, so a variety of antihistamines are acceptable. In these case loratadine (generic Claritin) is an affordable and effective choice. As the underlying Immune System Dysregulation (ISD) becomes more complicated then various other antihistamines can be considered.

Hydroxyzine (generic Atarax). This is commonly used in sufferers as this drug combines antihistamine and anxiolytic effects This agent is often used in PTSD sufferers, and because individuals with GDD experience various sources of stress, this drug may benefit them. We commonly use this antihistamine. Dosing ranges include: 10 mg three times a day, 25 mg twice a day, 25 mg three times a day.

Desloratadine (generic Clarinex) and Montelucast (generic Singulair) is a combination we have used in the past routinely. The description of the side effect of nightmares with Montelucast has stopped our routine use. However, this combination of antihistamines is a standard treatment for Mast Cell Activation Syndrome (MCAS). We opine that MCAS usually arises as a consequence of GDD and not necessarily a precursor,so when the co-existence of this is suspected, we use this combination. Montelucast is an antileukotriene, with Mast Cell membrane stabilization properties.

Standard is Hydroxyzine 5 mg in am, and Montelucast 10 mg at night.

Ketotifen: is an antihistamine with Mast Cell membrane stabilization properties. This agent then covers two useful properties. This needs to be compounded as it is not produced as a pill or capsule form in the USA. This agent again we will use in individuals with co-existent MCAS.

When to stop chelation:

When to stop chelation in general carries uncertainty. It is theoretically always possible to get more heavy metal out, but at some point this causes more harm than good. For Gd the principle is straightforward, and we apply the same principles for Lead and Cadmium. Two properties form the basis of that decision: 1) the patient describes they feel they are back to about 85% of their normal status, and 2) post-chelation Gd level (Lead, Cadmium the same considerations) is in the near normal range, so for Gd we use 3 mcg/ 24 hr (exception Prohance, Dotarem/Clariscan). In general the symptom perception is the dominant decision. The theory is that once an individual is at a 85% recovery level, they can carry out work and family obligations, and we allow the immune system to continue to calm down on its own. This more complete recovery may take as long as two years. For Gd, in general this is 5 chelation sessions for each GBCA injection. We monitor Lead and Cadmium as well with chelation.

We trial stopping chelation when the above two findings are met, which we term pausing chelation. Re-equilibration Flare always occurs at 1 month, if this Flare is minimal and then gets lower still by 3 months, we then consider chelation finished. If however Flare is moderate at 1 month and continues to escalate by 3 months, not enough chelation has occurred and we return to chelation. There are nuances to this decision.

Because of ongoing re-equilibration, patients may redevelop symptoms by 9- 12 months. Since now a lot of the Gd left has re-equilibrated back to soft tissue, generally a regimen of 3 additional chelation sessions is sufficient to achieve effective-cure.

Scientific principles of chelation: 1) the highest log stability constant chelator for the heavy metal in question available should be the primary treatment. and 2) it must be shown *in vivo* (in the person) to actually remove the metal.

Multimetal toxicity treatment.

Multimetal Toxicity

Multimetal toxicity is a common circumstance that arises once toxicity develops to one metal. Treatment for several of the heavy metals is identical, which makes treatment more straightforward in a number of settings.

Gd, Lead, Cadmium. These metals all have bone as the dominant durable reservoir. These metals all have relatively high log stability constant with DTPA: Gd (21), Lead (18.8), Cadmium (19) . This is a higher combination of stabilities than other chelators, hence DTPA is ideal to treat these 3. Also because of the bone dominance, they all require the step-wise chelation founded on le Chatelier's principle, with 3-4 week intervals between chelation.

Any of Gd, Lead, Cadmium in combination with Mercury, requires modification. Mercury is a complicated metal because it can be present in the body in a number of forms with different toxicities and different stabilities with various chelators. If Mercury is almost certainly present then trials of chelators on an individual basis should be tested. Start with DTPA (as DTPA is optimal for Gd, Lead, or Cadmium).pre- and post chelation 24 hr urine.

If no appreciable Mercury is removed, DMSA should be tried, obtaining 24 hr urines pre- and post-chelation. If DMSA removes significantly more Mercury, then a combination of DTPA and DMSA should be employed. How to perform this combination is a work in progress. There are positives and negatives for starting either one first:

Only DTPA:
Standard DTPA regimen (see Gd and Lead chapters).

Start with DMSA:
DMSA 250 mg TID. Three days in a row.
Ca-DTPA day 1/ Zn-DTPA day 2. One week after the third dose of DMSA.
Wait 2 weeks then repeat above.
A minimum repetition of 5 sessions.
The upside is this regimen would treat Mercury well, in the setting wjere Mercury is the principal symptomatic metal.
The downside of this regimen is that DMSA may result in damaging Gd redistribution.

Start with DTPA:
Ca-DTPA day 1/ Zn-DTPA day 2.
One week after DTPA
DMSA 250 mg TID. Three days in a row.

Wait 2 weeks then repeat above.

A minimum repetition of 5 sessions.

The upside is this regimen will remove Gd, Lead, Cadmium with no redistribution.

The downside is this regimen may redistribute Mercury.

Note that both of these patterns of combination can be tried at different times, and the patient's preference then used moving forward. The preference often is based on their symptoms of Flare reactions.

Other metals make treatment more complicated. Ancillary treatments that may be beneficial for a number of metals, may actually be detrimental for others. An illustrative example is the toxic form of chromium, hexavalent chromium. Although Hyperbaric Oxygen Treatment (HBOT) may have benefit as ancillary treatment for the bone depositing metals: Gd, Lead, Cadmium, the excess oxygenation would be very detrimental for Chromium. The management of Chromium toxicity is reduction therapy to convert the hexavalent (toxic) form to the trivalent (required for normal physiology) form. This can be achieved most simply with ascorbic acid, vitamin C. The use of HBOT would result in the opposite effect: oxidation rather than reduction, which would drive the equilibrium from physiologic trivalent to toxic hexavalent form.

Many of the patterns for regimens for treating Multimetal toxicity are yet to be formulated.

Radioactive metals:

The majority of the Actinide series metals (the next group of higher atomic number metals after the Lanthanides) are radioactive. This includes Plutonium and Uranium. It should be noted that Uranium-238, the most common isotope found in nature, has a half-life of 4.5 billion years, so it is effectively stable, and releases negligible radiation in a person's lifetime.

Radioactivity is defined by release of energy based on change in the atomic structure. There are 3 basic forms: 1) release of gamma rays without change in atomic number (atom stays the same element); 2) release of alpha particles: 2 protons and 2 nucleus (essentially a Helium nucleus) and a lower atomic number element created; and 3) Beta decay, which are described as Beta minus and Beta-plus. Beta-minus is more common, a neutron turns into a proton and releases an electron, and the electron is the energy release. The element created then becomes one position higher on the periodic table. Beta-plus is less common, a proton turns into a neutron and a positron is released as the emitted energy. The created atom is then one position lower on the periodic table.

The energy released by various particles is described as Linear Energy Transfer (LET). The LET for alpha particles is much higher than the other particles. The distance traveled in tissue is much shorter with higher energy particles. The LET for positron and electrons are much lower than that of alpha particles. Their LET is slightly higher than gamma- and x-rays. Gamma and x-ray are essentially identical in LET.

The LET reflects the ability of the particles/ energies to cause cellular damage. The cellular damage is oxidative stress, and the two effects of greatest concern are: i) direct tissue destruction from radiation, an immediate effect, and ii) the delayed effect of causing malignancies from the causation of DNA injury, specifically double-stranded DNA breaks. The malignancy causing potential of alpha particles >>> positrons, electrons> gamma rays, x-rays.

Early destructive damage is shown by skin reddening in low level exposures to aggressive destructive skin sloughing, blindness, bone destruction, and digestive tract sloughing. The risk of creating an immunogenic/toxic reaction from a radioactive metal is likely 1 in 10,000 as it is for stable metals. The risk of this then is a fraction of the risk of radiation damage, the latter which is 100%. Critical with radioactive metals is to remove them as quickly as possible, which is very different from the stepwise lengthy removal strategy with most stable heavy metals.

Various radioactive metals have different risks based on the particles they emit. Plutonium is an alpha emitter so risks of immediate tissue damage and cancer are significant. This is much greater risk of damage from Plutonium than most species of Uranium.

Radioactive heavy metal Treatment:

Current concept for removing radioactive metals is daily use of Zn-DTPA, on the basis that Zn-DTPA does not remove any appreciable amount of native netals. My preference would be to use Ca-DTPA since it removes a larger amount of heavy metals than Zn-DTPA. With Ca-DTPA, a strategy for native metal replacement would be needed. One approach is: 3 days Ca-DTPA, 1 day native metal iv infusion, performed repeatedly.

HOPO has been used for radioactive metal removal, and has the advantage of being administered orally. A combination of both chelators, and also various routes, including inhalation, could be structured as a multi regimen strategy.

Further Reading::

1.Martell AE, Smith RJ. authors.Title: Critical stability constants, Vol 6: Second Supplement. Plenum Press, NY, NY. 1992.

2.Semelka RC, Ramalho M. Gadolinium Toxicity and Current State of Knowledge and Expert Opinion. Investigative Radiology 2023; 58: 233-245.

3.Cheng YF, Zhao Yj, Chen C Zhang F. Heavy Metal Toxicity: Mechanism, Health Effects, and Therapeutic Interventions. Med-Comm 2025; 6: 245-258.

4. Domingo JL, Semelka RC. Gadolinium Toxicity:Mechanisms, Clinical Manifestations, and Nanoparticle Role. Archives of Toxicology 2025; 99: 3897-3916..

4. Fukuda S. Chelating agents used for plutonium and uranium removal in radiation emergency medicine. Current Medicinal Chemistry 2005; 12: 2765-2770.

CHAPTER

Eleven

GADOLINIUM.

Chapter 11. Gadolinium.

Background:

I have spent 10 years of my career, since 2015, focusing on the diagnosis and treatment of Gd toxicity, specifically GDD. Prior to that I have written major peer-reviewed articles on the subject of NSF beginning 17 years ago, since 2017, and on MR retention in the brain shown on MR images beginning 11 years ago, in 2014. I have written on acute hypersensitivity reactions (AHR) in textbooks for at least 30 years. So, I am the world authority on the subject of GDD toxicity. This chapter represents the distillation of that knowledge.The understanding of processes involved with other heavy metals stems from my knowledge gained on Gd. Of all heavy metals, the investigation into Gd comes closest to a controlled environment of science, as Gd has been administered at a known date, time and volume.

There are several distinctive features of Gd differing from other heavy metals, that render Gd toxicity assessment the closest to a controlled scientific setting. Gd exposure presently is confined to medical administration and not environment exposure, so the amount of Gd present in the body and the rate of administration are known. These are unknown with other metals with environmental exposure. In the same vein, since Gd is administered at a known time point with a short duration of incorporation, then symptoms and findings of toxicity are much more readily assignable to Gd, than is the case with other heavy metals. It is empirically obvious: symptoms and findings new to an individual arising immediately after, to within a couple of days, of Gadolinium Based Contrast Agent (GBCA) injection are symptoms due to Gd. The disease process caused by the presence of Gd that has resulted in persistent symptoms is termed Gd Deposition DIsease (GDD). GDD may originate up to 1 month post GBCA injection. In reality new symptoms can arise after that time point, especially if earlier on other symptoms of GDD have manifested. For the Gd toxicity arising in renal failure patients, Nephrogenic Systemic Fibrosis (NSF, a more specific term is Gadolinium-induced Systemic Fibrosis, GISF) new symptoms have been accepted as attributable to the disease if they are in the range of 2 months - 2 years. In recent years this time range has been expanded. The expansion on the earlier side of development, I interpret as reflecting that the patient has a combined toxicity of GDD-NSF or Acute Hypersensitivity Reaction (AHR)- NSF, and ofcourse AHR-GDD-NSF is a third possibility.

The treatment for GDD with DTPA chelation is the most appropriate treatment, beyond question, because we are essentially giving the individual the same type of chelate molecule that the Gd was administered with. No other heavy metal has been administered in chelated form, and yet chelation is accepted as the treatment for these metals. Of all metals, only Gd has been administered in a chelated form, and even more particularly, in a chelated form with the same type of chelator as the administered GBCA.

There is also a greater controlled setting for evaluating treatment success, as ongoing uncontrolled incorporation is absent with Gd, but present for other heavy metals.

Exposure source: Gadolinium Based Contrast Agents (GBCAs) used in MRI. The impact of higher content of Gd in the municipal water supply in regions with high density of MR machines (urban settings) is at present unknown.

Who are at risk: Approximately 1 in 10,000 individuals will develop GDD from a GBCA injection in MRI. There are additive risk factors described below.

Risk factors:

Risk factors that make developing disease more likely include: female 18-60 yrs, white race, multiple chemical sensitivity syndrome (MCSS), other chronic Immune Mediated Inflammatory Diseases (IMID), chronic infection (Lyme,COVID, COVID vaccine, varicella, Epstein Barr, CMV, etc), acute infections especially those requiring antibiotics, and other sudden perturbations of/ jolts to the immune system around the time of GBCA injection, including more serious events such as: recent severe infection with the addition of antibiotics as an additive factor; closely spaced CT study with iodine contrast to more simple events such as intense exercise. A common cluster of risk factors are: a white woman, 45 yrs of age, MCSS, and another pre-existing IMID causing Immune System Dysfunction (ISD). These are additive factors, in this example then the risk becomes 1 in 500 or more common. The MTHFR gene is present in 20-30%. A two-hit mechanism is common, but not always present, for susceptibility to develop GDD, such as the above described recent events prior to GBCA injection. The first hit disrupts normal action of the immune system, and the second hit is GBCA injection. This is distinct from the two-hit mechanism that creates the actual disease GDD, which is always present. The first hit is Gd disrupting the immune system, and the second hit is the intrinsic toxicity of Gd to cells.

Approximately 65% of sufferers are white women, 20% white men, and 15% of East Asian and Black race , women more common than men.

My current suspicion is that GDD may have a genetic cause, as is the case with another metal toxicity, Genetic Hemochromatosis. Genetic Hemochromatosis is also a white person disease, but even more exclusively as it is a Gaullic (French) genetic origin disease. GDD may also have an epigenetic cause,which is to say normal gene but with different behavior than standard for that gene. These possibilities are under investigation.

NSF may have the same gene/ epigenetic cause, but presumably with slight variance. NSF is observed in only 10% of individuals who have received the least stable GBCA, Omniscan. Low stability of the GBCA has the highest causative association with NSF. So immunological factors are also involved.

Complicating Factors:

Complicating factors are an overlapping set to risk factors, but are not identical. So risk factors like MCSS. is also a complicating factor. A person with MCSS may be sensitive to a whole range of drugs and chemicals so they require particular attention to all drugs used in their care, as the individual may be sensitive to them. This includes the type of steroid and type of antihistamines. Different from risk factors are complicating factors that are associated with higher retention of Gd, which includes surgeries that involve bones, or major surgeries in general. The more complicated the surgery the greater the complicating factor. Prior back surgery is a common complicating factor. These settings create the circumstance of more Gd going to aberrant bone, healing bone and to fibrosis in general. Most complicating factors do not mean that chelation will be ineffective, but that more chelations will be necessary. Our rule of thumb, for every GBCA 5 chelations are necessary. In the setting of severe/ extensive back surgery that number may be 10 rather than 5, or more.

My general recommendation is to postpone surgery till after 10 chelations have been performed, 5 chelations at the minimum. Basically so there is less Gd in the body that can be trapped in fibrosis or developing bone.

The more complicated the picture is of Immune Mediated Inflammatory Disease (IMIDs) and the resultant Immune System Dysregulation (ISD), the more prolonged the treatment will be. A beneficial aspect is the treatment for GDD with DTPA chelation and steroids/antihistamines does have a positive impact on most other IMIDs and sources of ISD.

All symptoms and findings may be GDD, and not everything is GDD.

These two apparently contradictory statements, reflect the common situation that two different thoughts need to be considered together. The most obvious way to solve this uncertainty is to start out considering that all symptoms are GDD. If by 10 chelation sessions (maybe up to 20 if the person has received > 10 GBCAs) there has been no change to certain symptoms, for example pelvic pain, then investigating at that point for an alternate additional condition, such as endometriosis in this example.

Molecular forms of Gd in the body:

Gd is present in many molecular forms in the body.This arises since Gd from many of the GBCAs undergo some level of disassociation from its administered ligand. This is frequently misdescribed as 'free' Gd, and this is erroneous because Gd is never free, but rapidly binds to other molecules. The most common forms of disassociated Gd, are re-bonded to phosphates and carbonates as small molecules, and bound into larger proteinaceous molecules.

A variable amount of Gd is maintained in its manufacture GBCA. In my opinion all of the injected Prohance and Dotarem/Clariscan remain chelated in their manufactured state. Gadavist, perhaps 20% to 50% from 1 month to 1 yr are bound to other molecules. Multihance perhaps 25% to 55% over that time frame. Magnevist 30% to 70%. Omniscan and Optimark 50% to 75%.

Another subject of debate is which of the molecular forms of Gd are the most symptomatic. Many experts consider that only disassociated Gd is symptomatic. Based on the fact that all GBCAs can cause AHR, my theory is that the most symptomatic forms of Gd are Gd bound to proteins and fully intact GBCA is also highly symptomatic.I base the latter on the fact that Dotarem/Clariscan and Prohance can cause both AHR and GDD even though they are likely still fully intact. One advantage of Gd bound to protein macromolecules is, that are more loosely attached and hence more removable from that molecule.

Symptoms:

Acute Hypersensitivity Reaction:

As suggested by the name, the symptoms of AHR are acute in onset and most last transiently. Symptom severity is classified as mild, moderate, severe.

The most common symptoms are mild, and these include skin reddening and hives. And head-ache, Incidence in the 1% range for all GBCA types.Nausea and vomiting are also common. The GBCAs that show protein-binding, Multihance and Eovist/ primovist, may show a slightly greater incidence of mild AHRs.

Throat swelling is a moderately severe symptom, and may require medical treatment.

Respiratory/lung symptoms are when an alert should be paid to the individual. Special attention to young to middle-aged women who are in good health. Anaphylactoid reaction is more likely to occur in them, and death can rapidly proceed if the catastrophic reaction is not controlled. Respiratory collapse and circulatory collapse are the feared outcomes. The explanation is that the mature and potent immune system in young females has the capacity to when dysregulated spiral out of control and initiate a Complement cascade. The complement system is a cluster of proteins that aide to the development of inflammatory reaction, which can be massive and life-threatening. Individuals with not fully developed immune systems (infants) and debilitated patients generally do not have an immune system powerful enough to mount a life-threatening reaction.

Steroids and antihistamines are generally used for severe cases of hives and throat swelling. The addition of epinephrine may be needed if severe reaction appears in progress, as well as cardiac drugs. Immediate call to emergency personnel is essential in severe AHR,

Death rate / mortality from AHR to GBCAs is reported as 1 in 300,000.

Gadolinium Deposition Disease:

GDD is primarily a persistent inflammatory/ toxic condition, caused by retention of Gd in the body. Gd stimulates an immune reaction/ IMID, which in turn facilitates the development of the substantial range of cellular and physiological toxic effects of Gd..

The most commonly experienced symptoms (Tier 1 symptoms) include the following:

cognitive impairment, skin pain, bone pain, muscle fasciculations, pins and needles sensations generally peripherally, handstand feet.

The causes for the symptoms reflect both the immunological effects and direct toxic effects of Gd, and also reflect that GDD is a multisystem, diffuse disorder.

Cognitive impairment reflects CNS involvement. This commonly is referred to as 'brain fog', but there is a whole range of CNS dysfunctions in this category, such as memory impairment, confusion, depersonalization, and Insomnia can also be included in this category.

Muscle fasciculations likely reflect both direct myocyte involvement and peripheral nerve involvement.

Skin pain and bone pain reflect direct local effects of Gd immunologic and toxic effects involving tissue resident memory T Cells, pro-inflammatory cytokines, and activation of TRPV1 ion channels. Skin pain is usually peripheral in hands and feet.

Pins and needles sensation in the hands and feet reflect small fiber neuropathy.

Tier 2 symptoms are commonly present in many subjects, but not as consistently as Tier 1. Many of these are direct organ action targeting nerves. These include: constricting head pain, imbalance/unsteadiness, hearing dysfunction, vision dysfunction, cardiac arrhythmias, digestive tract dysfunction, skin discoloration, and deep body burning.

Further description of some of these are worth mentioning because of the complexity.

Vision changes can involve multiple structures of the entire vision system. Double vision can result from extraocular muscle discoordination, floaters from Gd precipitates in the vitreous humor, flashing color due to optic nerve involvement and perhaps cortical brain.

Imbalance/unsteadiness. This likely reflects both the central nervous system (cerebellum), peripheral nerve, and muscle involvement. When severity is such that the individual is confined to a wheelchair, the recovery with treatment is uncertain.

Digestive tract dysfunction. Nausea and vomiting, which may be CNS and direct organ toxicity. Decreased digestive tract motility is the most problematic, gastroparesis and hypotonic small bowel and hypotonic colon are observed. Hypotonic small bowel can result in bacterial overgrowth in the small intestine (Small Intestinal Bacterial Overgrowth, SIBO or alternatively termed Small Bowel Intestinal Overgrowth, SBIO, I prefer SIBO).

Skin discoloration. Skin discolorations can be of many different colorations: yellow, red, black. These discolorations can be quite transient, lasting for a few days, or have longer duration: months to years. Dramatic transient black discoloration is the most striking and horrifying. Lower legs and feet are most affected by skin discoloration.

Tier 3 symptoms have been enumerated up to 100 symptoms. This reflects that Gd goes everywhere and can do just about anything. Hormonal changes of estrogen in women and testosterone in men are among the most noteworthy symptoms.

The above symptoms can arise acutely, and also are persistent. True chronic changes, meaning delayed onset and often relatively stable are observed.

Chronic symptoms/findings:

Skin: subcutaneous soft tissue thickening (doughiness) or loss. Soft tissue thickening is most common in the lower arms and hands. This is also the case with soft tissue loss. Soft tissue loss is also noted in the face especially in a distribution of the cheeks.

Skin wrinkling (cutis laxa). Uncommonly observed, the skin throughout the body may appear saggy and wrinkled. Effective treatment for wrinkling has yet to be elucidated. Similarly, although soft tissue thickening can improve with treatment, it is not clear if soft tissue loss can be regained,

Muscle wasting.

Teeth loss.

Mouth dryness and mucosal surface overgrowth.

Although the symptom complex of GDD is devastating, GDD is not associated with significant shortening of lifespan. Lifespan though is diminished, presumably by multiple years, as would be expected with any severe chronic disease.

Many of the cases of tooth loss likely reflect the insertion of Gd into the matrix of collagen in soft tissue, calcification in teeth, and bone in the teeth sockets and other bone structures. Gd becomes part of the architecture, but it is faulty and unstable. The faulty architecture can simply collapse, but also in the removal of the faulty architecture with chelation, this removal can also cause collapse. This means GDD itself causes these losses, but also chelation removal of Gd can cause this, the latter an unfortunate consequence of necessary treatment.

GBCAs in Pregnancy:

A large study performed in Ontario Canada that studied millions of pregnant women who underwent GBCA-enhanced MRI showed a higher rate of fetal loss and neonatal death than a matched population who did not receive a GBCA. The risk was relatively small. A reasonable recommendation at this time is to avoid GBCA administration, unless absolutely essential, in pregnant women. MRI **without GBCA** should be performed instead.Note that CT is also generally not recommended of the abdomen and pelvis in pregnant women due to the radiation risk of fetal injury and fetal cancer development.

GDD in children:

Gd toxicity in children, especially young children, merits particular description. As with autoimmune diseases, and IMIDs in general, Gd toxicity in young children is rare. My theory is because an intense reactogenic response of Deposition DIsease requires a mature immune system. Disease in young children generally manifests as a more pure Central Nervous System (CNS) disease, rather than a more broadly systemic disease as seen in adults. This reflects that the brain is still maturing and the neuronal axons are not fully myelinated, so they are more susceptible to injury. Seizures, delayed or ceased cognitive development, severe motor dysfunction all can occur and can be catastrophic. Generally preceding insults to the immune system like infections causing seizures increase the chances of childhood Gd toxicity. The incidence is uncertain but probably in the 1 in 100,000 range of children undergoing MRI.

Nephrogenic Systemic Fibrosis (NSF, Gadolinium -Induced Systemic Fibrosis, GISF):

NSF is a fibrogenic condition. The spectrum of symptoms reflect the diffuse fibrogenic process. Fibrosis, once mature, is also to date essentially irreversible.

Many of the most dramatic symptoms/ findings are of the lower legs and feet, and secondarily lower arms and hands. The dominance of this distribution is even more dramatic than that observed for GDD. This pattern reflects that blood has slower transit and pools in the lower legs and feet (hands not as much). The Gd that has been administered as a GBCA by intravenous injection is present in the slowly moving blood and deposits more and also removed less, because of this stagnation.

The most visually apparent findings are contractures of the lower legs and feet, which renders many sufferers wheelchair bound. Muscles of the hips, knees and feet are contracted by fibrosis.Hands are the next most common visually affected sites of contracture. Skin changes are often seen in the distal arms and legs, and these skin changes are shown as reddening and firm texture (woody).The symptoms and findings in NSF are chronic in nature and generally severe. Less severe forms most likely occur, and may escape detection.

All organ systems can experience fibrosis. Fibrosis of the chest wall musculature may be the most devastating, and likely the most common cause of death: pneumonia, due to the inability to cough up infective material well.. Death rate/ mortality from NSF is reported in the range of 50% but this would be a 5 year mortality figure.

Description of Gd in Humans and the Immune Reactions:

Gd distinguishes itself from all the other heavy metal toxic exposures in a few fashions: 1) Gd is used a medical tool, not an accidental exposure, 2) Gd is administered directly into the body by intravenous administration, whereas the others are by surface contact, most through the digestive tract, a few by cutaneous route, and a few others by inhalation into the lungs, and 3) is the only metal that is incorporated into the body as a chelate, which is therefore the exact mirror reflection of the principal treatment: chelation. Infact even the chelator is one that is used for GBCA manufacture.

There are 3 basic categories of toxicity::
1) Acute Hypersensitivity Reactions (AHR)
2) Gadolinium Deposition Disease (GDD)
3) Nephrogenic Systemic Fibrosis (NSF)/ Gadolinium Induced Systemic Fibrosis(GISF)

These entities can occur individually, but may also be composites of any grouping of them. The principal differences between these entities is the primary immune cell mediating the condition: AHR is mediated by MAST Cells (generally recognized theory), GDD by T cells , (principally tissue resident memory T cells (my theory)), and NSF by CD 34+ bone marrow cell infiltrates, the best recognized being circulating fibrocytes (generally recognized theory).

The time of onset of each of these conditions is driven by the predominant immune cell involved.

AHR can have immediate onset at time of injection to 1 day after. This is because MAST cell degradation of histamine and other inflammogens is rapid on exposure to a toxin.

GDD in a pure state has a time of onset 2 days to 1 month post GBCA injection, with various new symptoms continuing to announce themselves from 2 days to at least 3 months. At least 30% of GDD cases represent an AHR-GDD overlap, where the condition starts as a MAST cell reaction and converts to and persists as predominantly a T Cell reaction. The process of the immune reaction takes longer to develop for GDD. Antigen-presenting cells (example Dendritic cells), latch onto the foreign antigen (Gd, speciated into the administered GBCA or various recombinant species) and present the antigen to T cells, predominantly situated in lymph nodes. The T cells that are Gd-activated, then travel from lymph nodes to distribute throughout the body to all locations of Gd retention.

Although Gd is predominantly deposited in bone and skin, it is also distributed to all organs and tissues, hence Gd-activated T cells localize throughout the body. Surveillance positions for Gd are taken up by tissue resident memory T cells. Each organ has its own subtype of these resident T cells. My theory is the dominant Gd-reacting subtype is tissue resident memory T Cells.

GDD is the Gd version of Heavy Metal toxicity. It represents a persistent toxicity, and reflects a combination of immunologic / toxic reactions: a two-hit mechanism. The immunologic dysfunction is symptom-producing on its own, but it also permits the toxic properties of the heavy metal to occur. For Gd the proportion of the effects of immunogenicity (reactogenicity) and toxicity for symptom development are approximately 50/50. This ratio varies for each heavy metal.

NSF is a bone marrow cell reaction based disease. This means a collection of different types of immune cells, whose origin is the bone marrow. The best recognized is CD34+ circulating fibrocytes. This explains the late time of onset of disease, earliest at 2 months, and range of onset up to at least 2 years. NSF is generally observed in patients in renal failure who are on dialysis, that is renal failure category 5, with estimated Glomerular FIltration Rate(eGFR) < 15. Lesser levels of renal failure have also been observed with NSF. Earlier presentations of NSF have been reported. In my opinion these earlier cases represent a composite of NSF with AHR or GDD or both, in other words multiple cell lines of immune cells are involved.

AHRs, MAST cell reactions, are a common type of reaction. These reactions are most commonly observed for imaging contrast agents (Gd- based [MRI] and Iodine-based [CT]) and cancer drugs, but any type of drug can cause this. These are immediate onset reactions and most commonly are mild, resulting in hives. AHRs can however be massive, causing Complement cascades and Cytokine storms, termed anaphylactoid reactions, and have reported death rates: Gd generally reported as 1 in 300,000 administrations, and Iodine contrast 1 in 150,000. The higher safety of GBCAs I attribute to lesser volume of agent administered: GBCAs generally administered in 10 - 20 ml volume, and Iodine contrast 75- 150 ml volume. AHRs have been reported for Iodine contrast atleast since the 1960s, for Gd contrast atleast since the early 1990s. The general treatment for AHRs regardless of type of drug is with steroids and antihistamines, the most severe cases will require immediate epinephrine. Classically AHRs are of immediate onset and are short lived. So mild reactions of hives go away in days without treatment. When AHRs are massive they can cause death very quickly, if not recognized and treated quickly. I have focused on being very aware of young to middle aged women being at particular risk for anaphylactoid reaction and death if medical reaction is not swift enough. Once a person has developed an AHR reaction, this will repeat almost every time the antigen causing it is presented again to the individual.

Peanut allergy is in the category of AHR and I use the peanut reaction as a comparison for all allergies for heavy metals, even though the exact type of immune reaction differs, the concept is the same and easy to explain. The approach suggested for severe AHR to one brand of GBCA is to employ another brand next time. I currently prefer the approach of avoiding future GBCA injection altogether. One other unknown effect is a certain number of AHR cases do not respond to the standard antihistamine/steroids treatment, which is generally 1 day. It is not clear what then happens with these patients, as follow-up is generally absent in these reports. In my opinion,'failure of treatment' for AHR reflects that these individuals have transitioned from AHR to GDD.

A T Cell reaction, which GDD is an example, is also a very common type of allergy. This may be the most common type of allergy described for many drugs. This Is likely the most common reported reaction to Disease Moderating Anti-Rheumatic Drugs (DMARDS), such as Humira, Stellara, Cosentyx, etc. The ads for these agents on tv all state: 'if you are allergic to xxxx drug, don't take it'. This is our standard recommendation for GDD sufferers. T Cell based reactions, as in GDD, can be very devastating but do not appear to have the capacity to result in death. This is unlike MAST cell reactions, in which a small percentage can result in death. My opinion is that this reflects T cell based reactions and MAST cell based reactions follow different paths of escalation, where MAST cells can result in complement cascade and other associated immune pathways that can be lethal, but GDD does not. There may be an additional immune system dysfunction that occurs with GDD, which represents a communication error between antigen presenting cells (which are the cells that pick up the Gd in circulation and tissues) and the T cells that form the primary reaction and injury. The communication error being that the signal delivered is to **attack** Gd, rather than what happens in most individuals, those with Gadolnium Storage Condition which is **stay calm and carry on.**

Gd and other heavy metals persist in the body, which is unusual for drugs in general, so the source of reaction remains essentially permanently in the body, so this always has the result of causing toxic symptoms. The bone-dominant heavy metals (Gd, Lead, Cadmium) in particular remain for the lifetime of the individual. The primary treatment for T cell based inflammation of all types are steroids.A near unique property of the heavy metals compared to many other environmental toxins is they can be removed. The removal is achieved with chelation.

Bone marrow cell infiltrate reactions, of which NSF is an example, is generally the type of response the immune system generates when all other immune reactions have failed. This is the type of final reaction that Tuberculosis elicits, after other immune cells (for example neutrophils) have failed to combat the disease. Bone marrow cell infiltrates generally cause fibrosis surrounding the foreign antigen invader, encasing the entity to contain its negative effects. This fibrosis if exuberant then can be a cause for disease, as is the case with NSF. NSF is a disease of systemic fibrosis. The most often visual demonstrations are severe contractures of the distal legs and feet and secondarily distal arms and hands. The skin can be red and hardened with a woody texture. Many sufferers are confined to wheelchairs. Death is observed in about 1/2 of patients, and death most often is secondary to pneumonia. The chest wall muscles are involved, and the person's breathing and coughing are progressively diminished, so fluid no longer can be coughed out, and infection and death ensue. Bone marrow cel infiltrates are a relatively uncommon pattern of reaction especially when it appears to be the first line, which seems to be the case with NSF..

Of all the patterns of immune cell reactions, the pattern for NSF is the hardest to explain. AHRs with MAST cell reaction to antigens are very common. Similarly T cell reactions are quite common, this would be the primary form for all heavy metals. Immune reaction initiation with a bone marrow cell reaction is rare. Why patients with renal failure on dialysis are the group who experience this is also not understood. If retention of GBCA is the principal cause, and that NSF only occurs with lower stability linear GBCAs with a higher propensity for the Gd to disassociate (Omniscan, Optimark, Magnevist) why does this happen? All GBCAs in all individuals who have undergone GBCA injection have retention of Gd, so retention alone cannot explain this. Bone marrow cell infiltrate fibrogenic reactions must have an additional factor(s), either distinct chemicals, such as high phosphate or high uremia, bimetal heavy metal toxicity of Gd with Lanthanum. Lanthanum citrate is given to dialysis patients to lower phosphatemia, a particular defensive physiological reaction that individuals with advanced failure undergo, that creates the environment for NSF to develop, perhaps an epigenetic effect, and a gene may be related to NSF development.

It is also instructive to reflect on the history of Gd toxicity. Shawn Cowper, MD a dermatopathologist from Yale recognized the tissue findings of NSF in approximately 2000, but it was not till 2006 that Grobner a hemodialysis nephrologist in Austria made the association between the skin findings described by Cowper and MR Gd contrast (Omniscan first described).The second paper on the topic was written by another group of hemodialysis nephrologists, who were from Copenhagen, Denmark. It took 6 years to recognize the skin and contracture fibrotic entity was due to Gd from GBCAs. Also it was not Radiologists but a very specific group of nephrologists, hemodialysis physicians, who eventually recognized the connection, even though they saw all these patients. The literature on NSF was driven by hemodialysis nephrologists, so could not be ignored by Radiologists. Radiology had no control over what was published.

In contrast, approximately 1 in 10,000 individuals contract GDD after undergoing GBCA injection, and physicians of all specialties see these few patients. The chance of any one physician seeing even one patient with GDD, would be in the range of 1 per year. This relative rarity of GDD, was actually also confounded by the fact that physicians had been indoctrinated to believe that only patients with poor renal function developed Gd toxicity. Furthermore radiologists rarely see any patients, and even then only at the time of the imaging study, never in followup.These 3 factors served to obfuscate the existence of GDD. As incredible as it seems, many physicians to 2025 believe that only individuals with renal failure get a persistent disease from GBCA administration, mainly because NSF was the first reported entity.

The critical problem with failing to recognize that GDD exists is that it is a persistent disease, and even more importantly each successive GBCA injection makes the condition worse. This is the unethical part of failing to recognize GDD. Many individuals end up getting multiple additional GBCA injections with MRI to investigate what turns out to be GDD all along. The condition becomes worse with each additional GBCA injection, so failure to appreciate the existence of GDD, is not benign ignorance by physicians, it causes real harm to patients.

Prevention:

Many of the risk factors of GDD are out of control of the individual. Abrupt change in the status of the immune system around the time of GBCA injection is a significant risk factor to developing GDD I use this analogy: the immune system behaves in an orderly stepwise fashion to either calm down when presented with antigens that it should consider not a risk, and react to antigens that are a risk. An abrupt insult to the immune system then is like a tornado, and in a tornado it is easy to imagine that the immune system reacts adversely, when it should not, because everything is spiralling around, and it is difficult to keep a clear head when everything is in confusion.

. The most straightforward actions to **minimize an upset to the immune system include: maintain a low stress level; do not engage in intense physical activity within 1 week pre- and post-chelation, but mild activity is good (Goldilocks principle); have a normal to slightly increased level of hydration for 2 days before to 2 days after the GBCA injection at MRI; having an infection within 1 week prior to MRI, if possible postpone MRI till after an infection.** Kidney, breast and digestive tract infections have been associated with GDD development. Basically **avoid anything that can knock the immune system off its feet, even subtly**. Following the above will decrease the risk of developing GDD, but not eliminate it.

Treatment:

The basic treatment for heavy metal toxicity in general is chelation.This has been utilized for decades. The traditional agents used have been DMSA and EDTA, primarily because these were the agents available. Of all the heavy metal exposures, the only metal that is incorporated in humans as a chelate is Gd. Metals such as Lead and Mercury are not incorporated as chelates, so the chelation process involves attaching a foreign chemical, that they have never encountered before, to the metal. This may or may not work. In contrast Gd is administered as a chelate, which is the entire GBCA molecule, and is composed of Gd and a chelator. The chelator is termed a ligand in the context of manufacturing a GBCA. The chelator that is used is either identical or very close to the chelator used for chelation removal of Gd, DTPA.

The chelation process with DTPA for Gd is an exact mirror reflection of the considerations for manufacture of GBCAs.The difference is, **the primary role of the GBCA is to cause T1 relaxation in tissues for imaging**, so high stability by however means created is of paramount importance, for safety so no/minimal Gd is released. In short, increased T1 relaxation results in tissue brightening, and the most common reason to want this, is that cancers and inflammation become brighter than background tissue due to the effect of Gd. They then are much easier to see. For the chelator, the primary concern is also high stability so Gd remains attached to the chelator, but the **chelation process must have the ability to re-create a GBCA *in vivo*.**So the chelator has to be able to pick up Gd in physiological conditions of temperature and acidity in the human body. These constraints of *in vivo* (meaning in the living organism, in this case the person) creation are not present for the GBCA.

There are skeptics on the topic of using chelators to treat GDD, but what I find fascinating is that unlike Lead or Mercury, Gd is the only metal that has actually entered the body as a chelated metal, and even more striking, it is the same chelator, DTPA, which is a common chelator/ligand for MR GBCAs. How we remove Gd is then the actual mirror reflection of how it was administered.

The safety of DTPA is extrapolated from the data of the MR contrast agent Gd-DTPA, which is essentially Magnevist. Approximately 150 million doses of Magnevist have been given worldwide. No safety issue of the DTPA component of the contrast agent has ever been reported, and DTPA is the part of the molecule that makes the GBCA safe. It is the safe part of the GBCA. This level and quantity of safety data is essentially unparalleled with other chelators,those designed for chelating heavy metals, and at the highest echelon for prescription drugs.

The use of steroids and antihistamines is the standard of care for drug reactions. The chelation process by causing remobilization of heavy metals, creates the impetus to re-ignite the immune reaction to Gd, which is the Flare reaction. If the person is toxic from the metal remobilization of the metal has to cause a Flare. The combination of steroids and antihistamines have been used in at least 10s of millions of cases. These are the agents to reduce reactions, so the steroid resulting in reaction itself is exceedingly rare. The antihistamine however can cause a reaction of differing forms, so the antihistamine selected can be changed, if reactions to it occur..

How does chelation work: I use two analogies to describe how chelation works and the principle of the critical importance of stability constant.

The first is to consider chelation like the magnetic crane arcade game. A strong chelator is like a strong magnet in the crane. The stronger the magnet, the better able is the crane to pick up the magnet-bearing toy and transfer it to the exit shoot to deliver it to the player.This is the equivalent to Gd removal. A weaker magnet in the crane will release the magnet-bearing toy back in the pile. This is redistribution. The strength of the magnet in the toy is also important in this analogy. If both the crane and the toy have a strong magnet, then the crane will preferentially pick up the toy with the stronger magnet. In this analogy Gd has a very strong toy-magnet, compared to other cations like Calcium which is very weak. Gd is basically the strongest magnet in the entire collection of toys.

The second analogy is more complex and takes into account the 4 pieces to the puzzle of chelation and the final product of chelation, where positive and negative are attracted to each other.

The 4 pieces are: 1) the intrinsic negative electrical strength of the chelator, 2) the positive electric charge strength of the various cations that the chelator is administered to, 3) the positive electric charge strength of the heavy metal, and 4) the negative electric charge strength of whatever molecule the heavy metal is bound to. I imagine all these 4 combinations as magnets of various strengths on iron balls in a 1,000 channel pinball machine, where the pin balls are in pairs (negative bound to positive). The pinball pairs will bounce all around in the giant machine, but eventually most will end up in the pairings that have the strongest combination of electrical strength for both of them (one positive and the other negative). We can then take this analogy to the chelation setting. Calcium (Ca)-DTPA and Zinc (Zn)-DTPA bouncing around the body. With Ca-DTPA, Ca has a fairly low stability constant (low positive strength) with DTPA, on the order of 6, while Zn with DTPA has a stability of 12 (medium positive strength). So Zn-DTPA bouncing around will not exchange the Zn for the weaker positively charged: Calcium, Manganese, Magnesium, but will exchange Zn for the higher positive bond strength Gd, Lead, and Cadmium. Gd will dislodge from the weaker negative bond strength molecules that they are attached to in the body. Ca-DTPA having a weaker bond, DTPA will release Ca more readily, and will pick up some Mangenese, Magnesium, and Zn, but much of these native metals will be bounced off in favor of the much stronger bonding to Gd, Lead, and Cadmium. So millions of these magnetic ball pairs bouncing around, but the end result is the majority will end up with the strongest magnet pairs. So all 4 of these charge state particles need to be considered. In my opinion one addition to this game analogy, when DTPA encounters and even stronger negative charged molecule binding to the Gd (such as an intake molecule of Prohance and Dotarem/ Clariscan) it attaches to that complex and tugs it out of tissues into the circulation, which has been termed chaperoning in other chemical reactions.

The following is our standard regimen for Gd chelation:

DTPA Chelation Regimen

Three days before Chelation:

Stop taking personal supplements till 3 days after chelation.

Chelation Day One:

All injections below are given as a hand bolus at a medium rate, so drug injected over 10 seconds. Legs elevated on a footstool at 30 minutes time to facilitate Gd leaving the legs and traveling to the kidneys for excretion.

- 1 litre bag of iv normal saline with a 22 g or 24 g iv catheter. 1 port in iv line. (Full litre normal saline over 1 hour)
- iv Solumedrol as a split dose (62.5 mg) – (1/2 vial of solumedrol 125mg)
- Wait 10 minutes
- Split 1/2 dose of 5 ml vial Ca-DTPA (2.5 ml/ 0.5 g) iv bolus over 10 seconds.
- Wait 30 minutes
- Iv Solumedrol as a split dose (62.5 mg) – (1/2 vial of solumedrol 125mg)
- Wait 10 minutes
- Split 1/2 dose of 5 ml vial Ca-DTPA (2.5 ml/ 0.5 g) iv bolus over 10 seconds.

Chelation Day 2:

All injections below are given as a hand bolus at a medium rate, so drug in over 10 seconds. Legs elevated on a footstool at 30 minutes time to facilitate Gd leaving the legs and traveling to the kidneys for excretion.

- 1 litre bag of iv normal saline with a 22 g or 24 g iv catheter. 1 port in iv line. (Full litre normal saline over 1 hour)
- iv Solumedrol as a split dose (62.5 mg)
- Wait 10 minutes
- Split 1/2 dose of 5 ml vial Zn-DTPA (2.5 ml) iv bolus over 10 seconds.
- Wait 30 minutes
- Iv Solumedrol as a split dose (62.5 mg)
- Wait 10 minutes
- Split 1/2 dose of 5 ml vial Zn-DTPA (2.5 ml) iv bolus over 10 seconds.

Repeat above Chelation Regimen every 3 to 4 weeks for a total of 5 sessions for every GBCA injection.

Standard oral steroid regimen:

- **CHELATION DAY ONE:**

iv solumedrol usually sufficient

- **CHELATION DAY TWO:**

iv solumedrol usually sufficient

- **DAYS 1,2 AFTER CHELATION:**

Methylprednisolone (8mg)/atarax (25mg) in morning.
Methylprednisolone (8mg)/atarax (25 mg) at noon.
Methylprednisolone (8mg)/atarax (25 mg) in evening.

- **DAYS 3,4 AFTER CHELATION:**

Methylprednisolone (8mg)/atarax (25mg) in morning.
Methylprednisolone (8mg)/atarax (25 mg) in evening.

- **DAYS 5,6 AFTER CHELATION:**

Methylprednisolone (4mg)/atarax (25mg) in morning.

Methylprednisolone (4mg)/atarax (25 mg) in evening.

- **DAYS 7(+) AFTER CHELATION:**

Methylprednisolone (4mg)/atarax (25mg) in morning.
Atarax (25 mg) in evening.

Notes:

1. The first chelation session is generally performed with half the amount of chelator, in order to evaluate the level of Flare, and to accustom the patient to the Flare reaction. Above, full dose regimens often started chelation session 2.

2. If Flares continue beyond one week after Chelation Day One, Methylprednisolone can be continued at 8 mg or 4 mg for several additional days. Try not to exceed 4 additional days.This may be necessary after 21 days (with anticipated next chelation at 28 days after prior chelation), and is not uncommon for the 2-3 days prior to chelation to manage re-equilibration Flare.

3. Antihistamine Atarax. Generic Claritin (loratadine) is an acceptable alternative. Clarinex (5 mg) / Singulair (10mg) is an alternate antihistamine regimen, especial;ly if the individual may also have Mast Cell Activation Syndrome (MCAS) . Ketotaphen is also an option in concurrent MCAS.

4. The overall plan is to reduce steroids over the course of multiple chelations. Starting with dropping the amount of iv steroids to 1/2. Eventually eliminating iv steroids and use oral steroids 1 hour before, 1 hour after and in the evening on the days of chelation. The patient is also encouraged to drop the daily amount and number of days of steroid use, with the instruction to keep severity of Flare reaction at a level of 3-4/ 10 in severity.

5. Approximately 1/3 of GDD sufferers have the MTHFR gene variant so physiologically have decreased ability to methylate drugs, which means to modify them into their active form. This is a major reason that we use methylated steroids (methylpred-

nisolone) and also may select for desloratadine (Clarinex) which is the methylated form of this antihistamine.

Optimal timing for chelation should start at 3- 6 months after inception of GDD, and generally up to 1 year is ideal. Chelating within 10 days of GBCA injection would have the additional benefit of removing Gd before a full immune reaction to Gd has developed, so Flare reactions are not severe. In general we have recommended patients wait 3 months before starting chelation, for 2 reasons: 1) it avoids the highest alert status of immune cells, which is from 10- 75 days post GBCA injection, and is therefore the peak of intense Gd removal Flare. and 2) a number of patients will spontaneously resolve symptoms of GDD by 3 months. Probably at least 30% of individuals who received just 1 GBCA injection will resolve from GDD.Generally this improvement has already been noticeable by 60- 75 days. In subjects with early noticeable improvement continuing to watchful wait and not chelate may be appropriate. Near complete spontaneous recovery from GDD may take 2 years, using the watchful waiting approach. So one has to be prepared for that lengthy time period following this route. Spontaneous resolution occurs in about 30% of sufferers who just received 1 GBCA, and decreases to 15% after 2 GBCAs, 5% after 3, and extremely rarely occurs beyond 3.

GDD always gets worse with each additional GBCA injection, and often these GBCA injections are to investigate what turns out to be GDD all along. This is why early recognition by radiologists and MR facilities is critical. If GDD is recognized right away when it first starts, if the individual never gets another GBCA, 30% will recover with no specific treatment. The more GBCAs the person has received, the more chelations will be necessary. Generally the rule of thumb we use is for every GBCA the individual will require 5 chelation sessions.

EDTA had been attempted as a GBCA in the developmental phase of GBCA creation, but the bond between Gd and EDTA was too weak, too low stability, so it was never manufactured. I consider this the mirror reflection for chelation, if EDTA was too weak to be a GBCA, it is also too weak to be an effective chelator.

Response to chelation:

This has been described in detail in Chapter 9, but bears repeating here. The description of re-distribution is excluded here because this chapter pre-supposes that a strong chelator like DTPA has been used so negligible re-distribution would occur

There are 2 patterns observed when a high stability (> 20) chelator has been used. The presence of these Flares serves to confirm that the individual has GDD, if symptoms came on initially after GBCA injection:

1. **Heavy metal removal**.
2. **Heavy metal re-equilibration**. This represents le Chatelier's principle.:

Triphasic response to chelation

A triphasic symptom response to chelation has been well established in the peer-reviewed literature for Gd. Less experience with Lead and Mercury has nonetheless shown the same effect. Our opinion is that it is likely observed for many heavy metals.

With an effective chelator the following is observed:

Heavy metal removal Flare Days 0-5.

Period where improvement is observed Days 7-21.

Heavy metal re-equilibration Flare, Days 21-90, tailing off but continuing for 1 yr.

With subsequent chelations, Removal Flares decrease in length and severity, and the period of improvement increases and becomes more sustained. Re-equilibration Flare also diminishes, and this is the critical assessment to determine when to stop chelation.

It is worth noting that at times, Flares may unexpectedly be more intense farther along the course of a series of chelation sessions. The primary explanation is that although Gd may seem to come out of soft tissues, and later out of bone like sand trickling down an hour glass, more often, especially out of bone (re-equilibration phase) the Gd comes out more like icebergs breaking off a glacier, so coming out in chunks. So if a larger chunk of Gd comes out at some point, then it will stimulate more Flare. Other immune system effects may also be the cause for this variability, such as an intercurrent viral infection.

Supplements and Physical agents:

Ancillary treatment is often useful, in addition to the chelation regimen of DTPA chelation with steroids/antihistamines. .Of particular benefit to GDD includes substances with high anti-inflammatory properties: so turmeric, quercetin, spirulina, chlorella are the standards. Vitamin B (B complex), vitamin C can be important especially when removal of other additional heavy metals like Arsenic (vit B) and hexavalent Chromium (vit C) is necessary. Other supplements may be reasonable enough such as Sea Buckthorn. There are an enormous list of other supplements that could be used such as NAC, glutathione (oral or iv), they seem reasonable but I have not noticed benefits in patients.

Sauna does make a great deal of sense, perhaps conventional sauna is most appropriate.A natural defence mechanism is that sweat will eliminate a number of toxins, which includes heavy metals. This occurs though in a relatively small amount, nut any additional safe natural removal is helpful. **Caution:** Sauna should not be used if the individual has lost the ability to sweat. Hyperbaric Oxygen Therapy (HBOT) can be tried. Note this is contraindicated with hexavalent Chromium. Ozone I have not used, but may be of value.

Drugs: Low dose naltrexone (LDN) has been reported as effective. This we use. A number of sufferers have found benefit from CBD or THC. For particularly difficult cases the use of a potent DMARD or mTOR inhibitor like rapamycin may be a reasonable choice. Rapamycin at this point seems like the most reasonable strong immune modulating drug to consider. I would start at 1/2 the standard low dose. So this is starting at 5 mg. I do not have experience with this but this makes considerable sense to me.

Future Drugs: A future direction in drug use that may be especially helpful, serving to turn the key to the off position in reacting to Gd and perhaps other heavy metals are targeted JAK inhibitors and targeted blockers of a particular subtype of P2X protein.

GDD and Immune Mediated Inflammatory DIseases (IMIDs), and Immune System Dysregulation (ISD).

GDD is often the final IMID that enters the picture of ISD, and often then becomes the worst. So treatment of complicated scenarios should start with treatment of GDD.. Additional ancillary treatments for other IMIDs can be added concurrently, at times some spacing may be appropriate.

Treating mold toxicity concurrently with GDD makes sense in a number of individuals

Gd as a cause of other idiopathic Immune Mediated Inflammatory Diseases of unknown cause.

This has been discussed in chapter 9.. Gd-caused Fibromyalgia is likely a common situation. Also it is uncertain, but I suspect that a number of cases of prolonged COVID or COVID vaccine toxicity may partly actually reflect GDD, if the individual also had a GBCA investigating symptoms of these entities.

Outcomes:

Isolated GDD does have a cure rate approaching 100%, when there are no significant risk factors, complicating factors, IMIDs, and few GBCA injection. In general, if enough DTPA chelations are performed then near cure rates are in the 90 - 95% range for most individuals regardless of complicating factors. About 5% of individuals do not respond appreciably to DTPA chelation, which at the present time I interpret that another pre-existing IMID shows no response to chelation and blocks or overshadows any response of GDD to chelation. I use the term near cure as I consider it most likely that even well treated GDD becomes like other conditions that have a persistent nidus or kernel remaining in the body. This persistent kernel can re-ignite symptoms of GDD at any time, most commonly in the setting of stress. This may seem distressing to learn this, but we all possess other entities that can cause this same situation if they persist in our bodies they can re-activate. Common agents that are like this are Herpes Virus, CMV virus, Varicella virus, that at times of stress symptoms will express themselves. This re-activation can also be used as a positive. It informs the individual that they have been under too much stress and should calm down. So this can be a mechanism to enact stress reduction. The other positive worth mentioning, is that when a person has GDD they are now forced to eat a healthy diet and engage in regular exercise to counteract the disease. So for many this may carry the prospect of a longer and healthier life. When possible look for the silver lining in bad events. Like GDD.

Caution: Use new supplements / treatment methods as often or best as possible one at a time, and start at low

amount and work up. The immune system of GDD and other heavy metal toxicity sufferers is dysregulated and may respond poorly or with severe reactions to new things, even if it works well for others. With ISD, a person's immune system can respond erratically and unpredictably to various exposures. I do not recommend combining in a short interval other methods with DTPA chelation, space them out, usually 1 week apart.

Further Reading::

1.Semelka RC, Ramalho M. Gadolinium Toxicity and Current State of Knowledge and Expert Opinion. Investigative Radiology 2023; 58: 233-245

2.Cheng YF, Zhao Yj, Chen C Zhang F. Heavy Metal Toxicity: Mechanism, Health Effects, and Therapeutic Interventions. MedComm 2025; 6: 245-258.

3. Domingo JL, Semelka RC. Gadolinium Toxicity:Mechanisms, Clinical Manifestations, and Nanoparticle Role. Archives of Toxicology 2025; 99: 3897-3916.

4. Murata N, Murata K, Gonzalez-Cuyar LF, et al. Gadolinium Tissue Deposition in Brain and Bone. Investigative Radiology 2016; 51: 671-678.

5. Martell AE, Smith RJ. authors.Title: Critical stability constants, Vol 6: Second Supplement. Plenum Press, NY, NY. 1992.

6. Coimbra S, Rocha S, Sousa NR. Toxicity mechanisms of Gadolinium and Gadolinium-Based contrast agents. 2024. In J Mol Sci; 25: 4071- 4087.

CHAPTER

Twelve

LEAD

Chapter 12. Lead

Exposure sources: There is a long history of the use of Lead by humans. Exposure to Lead increased dramatically in humans after the Industrial Revolution and the pollution generated by industry. The highest human levels in the developed/ developing nations occurred in the early to mid 20th century primarily from Lead in gasoline. In the US lead was progressively removed from paint in the 1950s and from automobile gasoline in the 1970s. Nonetheless even to the present time Lead is found in many products, including baby food and tampons. As Lead is present in essentially all North Americans, a consistent source of Lead is from fetal exposure to maternal circulation. Presently, Lead contamination in Lead pipes delivering the municipal water supply to older communities is both the largest and most worrisome source of Lead. Flint Michigan is the most recognized community for this, and for the neurotoxicity effects in children.

Who are at risk: There is not a clear gender or race risk for developing Lead toxicity/ Deposition Disease. It may be that it parallels that observed for Gd, that women are at greater risk for toxicity. Children exposure is of greatest concern, especially for acute, large dose exposures.

Symptoms: Different from Gd, where the dosages and time of acquisition for Gd is clearly defined, intake of Lead is often more insidious and of very long duration,although acute massive exposure can occur.

The common symptoms of Lead toxicity are:

1. abdominal pain and cramping,
2. fatigue,
3. general weakness,
4. headaches,
5. irritability/ mood changes
6. cognitive impairment, typically memory impairment, difficulty concentrating .
7. depression
8. joint pain
9. muscle pain
10. loss of appetite, weight loss
11. metallic taste
12. high blood pressure
13. seizures, encephalopathy, especially in young children with very high level exposure.

It is noteworthy that although a large quantity of Lead is deposited in bone, Lead Toxicity- sufferers generally do not describe sharp bone pain, as described in GDD sufferers and Cadmium toxicity sufferers.

Lead in children:

Childhood exposure to Lead requires specific attention. Lead toxicity is less common in children than in adults, as is the case with auto-immune diseases. This belies the immunologic/ toxic two-hit mechanism of the effective toxicity of Lead. The central and peripheral nervous systems in children are still in the maturation process of myelination of axon sheaths. Axon sheaths coat the axons, to protect and speed neural connections. Axons are the connecting wires extending from neurons to other neurons and other cells. In the central nervous system (CNS) the myelination process is accomplished by oligodendrocytes and in peripheral nerves by Schwann cells. The immature development status of myelination renders the CNS and major peripheral nerves especially sensitive to toxic injury from Lead. Therefore in children Lead toxicity primarily affects the CNS, more so than in adults, and the damage can be profound and at times catastrophic. Seizures and delayed/blocked cognitive development are features of severe childhood toxicity.

Avoidance:

Avoidance is not possible with Lead, which is also the case with the majority of heavy metals. Therefore the approach is minimization of exposure. Among all heavy metals, the US government has been the most pro-active in decreasing exposure to the population as evidenced by legislation to remove lead from paint and gasoline. An important role still rests with the individual to pay attention to health reports of lead presence in products, such as the findings of increased lead in certain brands of baby food, tampons, and most recently packaged meat products.The amount of lead in products is important. Armed with this information individuals can decide what they will do.

Detoxification: Because Lead is so pervasive and disease so insidious, it is particularly important to pay close attention to an overall detoxification program. This starts with eating a healthy, balanced diet, and paying attention to news reports regarding the presence of an abnormally high lead content in various food and consumer products. The reader is directed to the chapter on detoxification for a more detailed discussion of a detoxification program.

Treatment:

Treatment for Lead toxicity /Lead-Deposition Disease is with chelation. Traditional chelation has used DMSA, EDTA, or a combination of both. Based on stability, DTPA is mildly superior to EDTA, DTPA 18.8, EDTA 18.1, DMSA is 16. So for pure Lead-DD EDTA is generally effective, but DMSA is not as recommended because the stability constant is too low..

Our preference is to use DTPA rather than EDTA, as it is more stable, has more affinity, for Lead, approximately 80 times, and hence will result in less undesirable Lead redistribution. EDTA is an acceptable alternative. If the individual has multimetal toxicity including Gd and/or Cadmium, DTPA would be strongly advised because of its significantly higher stability for these two metals, which are the two other bone-dominant durable reservoir metals. This also means that chelation intervals in the 3-4 week range are more ideal than 1 week, to allow for more re-equilibration of Lead from bone back to soft tissues, for much more effective removal. Lead chelation is never a one time event, because of the dominant bone retention. A minimum of 5 chelation sessions spaced 3-4 weeks apart is recommended. This accomplishes the stepwise reduction of total body Lead content through le Chatelier's principle.

Below is the recommended chelation regimen. EDTA can be substituted in for DTPA, and can use the identical regimen.

Chelation Day One:

All injections below are administered as a hand bolus at a medium rate, so drug injected over 10 seconds.

- 1 litre bag of iv normal saline with a 22 g or 24 g iv catheter. 1 port in iv line. (Full litre normal saline over 1 hour)
- iv Solumedrol as a split dose (62.5 mg) – (1/2 vial of solumedrol 125mg)
  - Wait 10 minutes
- Split 1/2 dose of 5 ml vial Ca-DTPA (2.5 ml/ 0.5 g) iv bolus over 10 seconds.
  - Wait 30 minutes
- Iv Solumedrol as a split dose (62.5 mg) – (1/2 vial of solumedrol 125mg)
  - Wait 10 minutes.
- Split 1/2 dose of 5 ml vial Ca-DTPA (2.5 ml/ 0.5 g) iv bolus over 10 seconds.

Chelation Day 2:

All injections below are administered as a hand bolus at a medium rate, so drug is injected over 10 seconds.

- 1 litre bag of iv normal saline with a 22 g or 24 g iv catheter. 1 port in iv line. (Full litre normal saline over 1 hour)
- iv Solumedrol as a split dose (62.5 mg)
  - Wait 10 minutes
- Split 1/2 dose of 5 ml vial Zn-DTPA (2.5 ml) iv bolus over 10 seconds.
  - Wait 30 minutes
- Iv Solumedrol as a split dose (62.5 mg)
  - Wait 10 minutes

- Split 1/2 dose of 5 ml vial Zn-DTPA (2.5 ml) iv bolus over 10 seconds.

Repeat above Chelation Regimen every 3 to 4 weeks for a total of 5 sessions for every GBCA injection.

Standard oral steroid regimen:

- **CHELATION DAY ONE:**

iv solumedrol usually sufficient

- **CHELATION DAY TWO:**

iv solumedrol usually sufficient

- **DAYS 1,2 AFTER CHELATION:**

Methylprednisolone (8mg)/atarax (25mg) in morning.
Methylprednisolone (8mg)/atarax (25 mg) at noon.
Methylprednisolone (8mg)/atarax (25 mg) in evening.

- **DAYS 3,4 AFTER CHELATION:**

Methylprednisolone (8mg)/atarax (25mg) in morning.
Methylprednisolone (8mg)/atarax (25 mg) in evening.

- **DAYS 5,6 AFTER CHELATION:**

Methylprednisolone (4mg)/atarax (25mg) in morning.
Methylprednisolone (4mg)/atarax (25 mg) in evening

- **DAYS 7(+) AFTER CHELATION:**

Methylprednisolone (4mg)/atarax (25mg) in morning.
Atarax (25 mg) in evening.

Notes:

1. The first chelation session is generally performed with half the amount of chelator, in order to evaluate the level of Flare, and to accustom the patient to the Flare reaction. Above, full dose regimens often started chelation session 2.

2. If Flares continue beyond one week after Chelation Day One, Methylprednisolone can be continued at 8 mg or 4 mg for several additional days. Try not to exceed 4 additional days.This may be necessary after 21 days (with anticipated next chelation at 28 days after prior chelation), and is not uncommon for the 2-3 days prior to chelation to manage re-equilibration Flare.

3. Flares are generally not as intense as with Gd, so decreasing the amount of steroids used as iv and oral drugs can be more rapidly decreased.

4. Antihistamine Atarax. Generic Claritin (loratadine) is an acceptable alternative. Clarinex (5 mg) / Singulair (10mg) is an alternate antihistamine regimen, especial;ly if the individual may also have Mast Cell Activation Syndrome (MCAS) . Ketotaphen also an option in concurrent MCAS.

5. Approximately 1/3 of GDD sufferers have the MTHFR gene variant, this may also be the case in Lead toxicity sufferers, so physiologically have decreased ability to methylate drugs, which means to modify them into their active form. This is a major reason that we use methylated steroids (methylprednisolone) and also may select for desloratadine (Clarinex) which is the methylated form of this antihistamine.

Outcomes:

Chelation with DTPA is very effective for removing Lead, and results are generally very good. Results in children may be only fair if significant CNS injury has occurred. Unlike Gd, continued Lead incorporation is expected, so more long term methods to minimize continued Lead exposure are required. This may include routine consumption of an effective oral chelator long term. To date, an oral form of DTPA or similar agent has not yet been developed. Oral EDTA may be adequate. Oral HOPO could be used for this purpose once it becomes FDA approved.

Further Reading::

1. Lanphear B. Lead Poisoning. New England Journal of Medicine 2024; 390: 501-513.

2 .Martell AE, Smith RJ. authors.Title: Critical stability constants, Vol 6: Second Supplement. Plenum Press, NY, NY. 1992.

CHAPTER

Thirteen

CADMIUM.

Chapter 13. Cadmium.

Exposure Sources: Contaminated water, rice and shellfish are the most recognized sources. Battery manufacture workers and smoking are additional sources.

Who are at risk:: No specific demographics beyond exposure.

Retention sites: 70% retained in bone. 30% in kidneys.

Symptoms:

The most recognized symptom description is "Itai-Itai" in Japanese, which is "it hurts, it hurts" . This refers to the severe bone pain sufferers often experience.

The common symptoms are:

1. Bone pain.
2. Renal failure from kidney accumulation.
3. Weakness
4. Lung disease from smoking or inhalation in battery factory workers

Avoidance: Avoid eating shellfish if Cadmium is elevated in native 24 hr urine.

Detoxification: Standard detoxification as described in Detoxification chapter.

Treatment:

The traditional treatment for Cadmium toxicity is chelation therapy. The optimal treatment is with DTPA as it has both the highest stability constant for Cadmium (19) among all available chelators, and is well excreted by the kidneys. The chelation technique described for Gd is also ideal for Cadmium, since Cadmium is also a bone-deposition-dominant heavy metal condition, the same strategy for Gd and Lead of 3 week intervals between chelation sessions is recommended to optimize re-equilibration based bone Cadmium removal. Cadmium is commonly elevated along with Gd and Lead.

DTPA Chelation Regimen

Three days before Chelation:

Stop taking personal supplements till 3 days after chelation.

Chelation Day One:

All injections below are administered as a hand bolus at a medium rate, so drug injected over 10 seconds.

- 1 litre bag of iv normal saline with a 22 g or 24 g iv catheter. 1 port in iv line. (Full litre normal saline over 1 hour)
- iv Solumedrol as a split dose (62.5 mg) – (1/2 vial of solumedrol 125mg)

\- Wait 10 minutes

- Split 1/2 dose of 5 ml vial Ca-DTPA (2.5 ml/ 0.5 g) iv bolus over 10 seconds.

\- Wait 30 minutes

- Iv Solumedrol as a split dose (62.5 mg) – (1/2 vial of solumedrol 125mg)
- Wait 10 minutes
- Split 1/2 dose of 5 ml vial Ca-DTPA (2.5 ml/ 0.5 g) iv bolus over 10 seconds.

Chelation Day 2:

All injections below are given as a hand bolus at a medium rate, so drug in over 10 seconds.

- 1 litre bag of iv normal saline with a 22 g or 24 g iv catheter. 1 port in iv line. (Full litre normal saline over 1 hour)
- iv Solumedrol as a split dose (62.5 mg)
- Wait 10 minutes
- Split 1/2 dose of 5 ml vial Zn-DTPA (2.5 ml) iv bolus over 10 seconds.
- Wait 30 minutes
- Iv Solumedrol as a split dose (62.5 mg)
- Wait 10 minutes
- Split 1/2 dose of 5 ml vial Zn-DTPA (2.5 ml) iv bolus over 10 seconds.

Standard oral steroid regimen:

- **CHELATION DAY ONE:**

iv solumedrol usually sufficient

- **CHELATION DAY TWO:**

iv solumedrol usually sufficient

- **DAYS 1,2 AFTER CHELATION:**

Methylprednisolone (8mg)/atarax (25mg) in morning.
Methylprednisolone (8mg)/atarax (25 mg) at noon.
Methylprednisolone (8mg)/atarax (25 mg) in evening.

- **DAYS 3,4 AFTER CHELATION:**

Methylprednisolone (8mg)/atarax (25mg) in morning.
Methylprednisolone (8mg)/atarax (25 mg) in evening.

- **DAYS 5,6 AFTER CHELATION:**

Methylprednisolone (4mg)/atarax (25mg) in morning.
Methylprednisolone (4mg)/atarax (25 mg) in evening.

- **DAYS 7(+) AFTER CHELATION:**

Methylprednisolone (4mg)/atarax (25mg) in morning.
Atarax (25 mg) in evening.

Notes:

1. The first chelation session is generally performed with half the amount of chelator, in order to evaluate the level of Flare, and to accustom the patient to the Flare reaction. Above, full dose regimens often started chelation session 2.

2. If Flares continue beyond one week after Chelation Day One, Methylprednisolone can be continued at 8 mg or 4 mg for several additional days. Try not to exceed 4 additional days.This may be necessary after 21 days (with anticipated next chelation at 28 days after prior chelation), and is not uncommon for the 2-3 days prior to chelation to manage re-equilibration Flare.

3. Antihistamine Atarax. Generic Claritin (loratadine) is an acceptable alternative. Clarinex (5 mg) / Singulair (10mg) is an alternate antihistamine regimen, especial;ly if the individual may also have Mast Cell Activation Syndrome (MCAS) . Ketotaphen is also an option in concurrent MCAS.

4. The overall plan is to reduce steroids over the course of multiple chelations. Starting with dropping the amount of iv steroids to 1/2. Eventually eliminating iv steroids and use oral steroids 1 hour before, 1 hour after and in the evening on the days of chelation. The patient is also encouraged to drop the daily amount and number of days of steroid use, with the instruction to keep severity of Flare reaction at a level of 3-4/ 10 in severity.

5. Approximately 1/3 of GDD sufferers have the MTHFR gene variant, it is unknown if this is also the case with Cadmium sufferers. It may be prudent to also use methylated drugs:methylated steroids (methylprednisolone) and also may select for desloratadine (Clarinex) which is the methylated form of this antihistamine.

Outcome:

Outcome for DTPA chelation for Cadmium toxicity that is less than 5 years, should be good. There is no published data currently available.

Further Reading::

1..Cheng YF, Zhao Yj, Chen C Zhang F. Heavy Metal Toxicity: Mechanism, Health Effects, and Therapeutic Interventions. MedComm 2025; 6: 245-258.

2. Charkiewicz AE, Omeljaniuk WJ, Nowak K, Garley M, Nilinski J. Cadmium Toxicity and Health Effects-A Brief Summary, Molecules 2023; 28: article 6620.

3. Martell AE, Smith RJ. authors.Title: Critical stability constants, Vol 6: Second Supplement. Plenum Press, NY, NY. 1992.

CHAPTER

Fourteen

MERCURY.

Chapter 14. Mercury.

Mercury is a more complicated heavy metal than many of the others, as it is incorporated into humans in different forms: inorganic Mercury and a variety of organic subtypes with the most common toxic form being methyl Mercury.

Sources:

Inorganic Mercury: primary sources are dental amalgums, older product thermometers, industrial exposure.

Organic Mercury: the most detrimental common form is methyl Mercury and the most common source is from eating large predatory fish: Tuna, salmon, shark, swordfish.

The classic historical description of Mercury toxicity is Mad Hatter's Syndrome. Hat makers in the 18th and 19th centuries used mercury nitrate in the felting process. 'Mad' came from the very unusual and erratic behavior and thought patterns that sufferers manifested. The most famous example of Mercury toxicity is that of Emperor Chin, the first emperor of China,. In his drive to live long he instructed his physicians to provide him with life prolonging treatments. They gave him inorganic Mercury orally, thinking that its unusual property of being a thick fluid at room temperature that forms beads and coalesces, must somehow be good for you. The first emperor died relatively young and very crazy from the Mercury toxicity.

The two Mercury sources of greatest public interest are inorganic mercury in dental amalgums and organ mercury in large fish species. The risk for Mercury toxicity from dental amalgums is generally considered low for the majority of individuals.

Who are at risk: Generally exposure alone is the most common underlying cause for Mercury toxicity, not specific age or gender. Although the risk concern is greatest for pregnant women and young children.

Symptoms: The symptoms that Mercury causes are primarily neurological, affecting both the CNS and peripheral nerves.

1. numbness and tingling, especially hands and feet. Peripheral nerves .Small fiber neuropathy.
2. tremors, coordination problems. CNS and peripheral nerves
3. cognitive impairment, memory loss, difficulty concentrating. CNS effect.
4. severe cognitive disorders; paranoia, psychotic-type thinking. CNS effect.
5. mood swings CNS effect
6. instability, difficulty walking.CNS and peripheral nerves
7. muscle weakness and atrophy. CNS and peripheral nerves

The symptoms most distinctive for Mercury compared to other heavy metals are the more bizarre cognitive issues of paranoia and psychotic-like state.

Storage sites:

1. Brain.
2. Fatty issue
3. Kidneys
4, Liver, minimal.

Avoidance: If Mercury level is high on native urine testing, the first approach is to stop eating large predatory fish, such as tuna and swordfish.

Treatment:

Inorganic Mercury has an extremely high stability with DTPA, 26, and considerably higher than with EDTA (18), and DMSA (14), however it is not the most toxic or common form. DTPA then would be the optimal chelator if dental amalgums are the concern.

Methyl Mercury is the most worrisome of the common forms of Mercury. The stability constants are : DMSA (16), EDTA (10-12) and DTPA (10-12). DMSA is the current agent of choice for chelation, although an agent with stability closer to 20 would be preferred.

DMSA Conventional treatment:

250 mg three times per day. Often an approach that has days on and days off. Such as 3 days on, 3 days off.

We recommend a more modern approach for performing Mercury treatment:

Obtain 24 hr urine prechelation. If Mercury is elevated, but also Lead, possibly also Cadmium, and Gd.

Perform 1 g Ca-DTPA bolus administration, as described for Gd, Lead and Cadmium as well. Recommend iv steroid use concurrent with chelation The Flare reaction if the person has Mercury toxicity is often intense paranoia and psychotic-like behavior that can be very problematic. The sufferer will benefit from a companion, as the bizarre behavior may render them incapable of reasoning, and unable to continue to undergo chelation treatment.

If Mercury also shows substantial increase in urine content post DTPA, using this chelator alone may be sufficient.. If the increase is not substantial but Mercury toxicity remains of clinical concern, then a regimen including oral DMSA and iv DTPA is recommended. These chelators should be staggered.

Alternate treatment regimen considering teeth amalgams :

Ca-DTPA day 1/ Zn-DTPA day 2. Wait one week. 3 days of DMSA 250 mg three times per day. One week's pause. repeat Ca-DTPA day 1/ Zn-DTPA day 2. When multiple metal toxicity is suspected, 5 cycles of this approach would be the minimal therapy.

Re-equilibration Flare is always the symptom to look for to determine when treatment is sufficient. With trial stopping, the re-equilibration Flare should be minimal and progressively decline over a 4 month period.

Possible treatment method:

Emeramide is a newer chelating agent that has an apparent positive effect for Mercury removal, typically given orally. Typical dosages are 100-300 mg, once or twice per day. A recommended regimen to start is 100 mg twice a day for 3 days, break for 3 days, then repeat.

I always recommend doing a provoked test with an agent where the effectiveness is uncertain. To see if Emerimide is actually working to remove Mercury. Obtain unprovoked 24 hr urine within 3 days of chelation. Take 300 mg of Emeramide, wait 1 hour and repeat a 24 hour urine test. If Mercury level goes up four fold or more, then continue using Emeramide.

Toxic mechanisms of Mercury.

The principal toxic effects of Mercury have been attributed to its binding effect to sulfur groups in proteins. This binding impairs/ destroys the ability of these proteins to function. This has been considered the explanation for the neurological symptoms. The most recent research has focused on the disruption of surface membrane binding of cells with focus on the protein Besigin (CD147). The cell membrane binding disruption affects many different chemicals, one of which is lactate. Lactate presence in cells also comports with the general concept of the Goldilocks principle: it has to be in the right amount, and in the right amount for various functions, which varies.

In concurrence with a main focus in this book, the effect of Immune System Dysfunction induced by Mercury has been reported.

Outcome:

As Mercury appears in various forms, and the damage in primarily to nerves, central and peripheral, treatment and recovery are more variable. Also the effect of other metal toxicities is often present, with the most common additional metal is Lead. A chelator with higher stability for methyl Mercury than presently available would be beneficial.

Bibliography:

1. Wilson MC, Meredith D, Manning Fox JE, et al. Basigin (CD147) is the target for organomercurial inhibition of monocarboxylate transporter isoforms 1 and 4: the ancillary protein for the insensitive MCT2 is EMPIGIN (gp70). Journal of Biological Chemistry 2005; 280: 27213-27221.

2.Bjorklund G, Peana M, Dadar M, et al.Mercury-induced Autoimmunity: Drifting from Micro to Macro Concerns on Autoimmune Disorders. Clinical Immunology 2020; 213: article 108352.

CHAPTER

Fifteen

ARSENIC.

Chapter 15. Arsenic.

Exposure sources:

1. Rice
2. Contaminated water.
3. Occupational exposure in mining, smelting.
4. Shellfish
5. Pesticides and rodenticides
6. Classic nefarious poison.

Arsenic was added to chicken feed to promote growth and prevent infection, This was stopped in the USA in approximately 2000. The administration of arsenic into pesticides has been phased out over the last 2 decades. These are positive examples of attention to potential sources of heavy metal toxicity.

Who is at risk: Individuals with a high level of exposure.

Symptoms:

Acute Disease:

1. Seizures, convulsions, respiratory distress, severe gastrointestinal distress. Foaming at the mouth reflects the combination of convulsions and severe respiratory distress. (acute, and severe chronic).
2. Liver and kidney injury/ failure.

Chronic Disease:

1. skin pigmentation and thickening
2. gastrointestinal:nausea, abdominal pain
3. Neurological: peripheral numbness and tingling
4. Garlic smell on breath.

Avoidance: Minimization of exposure is achievable.. Brown rice contains more Arsenic than white rice, so avoid brown rice. The explanation is Arsenic accumulates in the outer layer of rice (brown rice is rice with outer layer still present). Avoid eating shellfish.

Detoxification:

B complex vitamins are important. Standard detoxification approach.

Treatment:

There are multiple forms of inorganic and organic species of Arsenic. The inorganic forms are generally more toxic than the organic forms. Organic forms are often found in seafood. Organic arsenic is less toxic because it is more easily metabolized and removed.

The standard chelator used for Arsenic is DMSA at the present time. A reasonable protocol is 250 mg three times a day for 3 days, then 3 days off, and repeat. Five sessions of this may be a reasonable approach.

None of the standard chelators are that effective, as reflected by the stability constant. The stability with DMSA is 12, with EDTA and DTPA 8-10. So DMSA is currently the best available chelator, but is still only fair.

24 urine pre- and post-chelation is a useful approach to assess the effectiveness of a chelator. DTPA may also be effective, and 24 hour urine measurements would determine its effectiveness. The variability may stem from the type of Arsenic incorporated.

Niacin, vitamin B3 and Folate, vitamin B9, may help with methylation, reducing the toxicity of some species of Arsenic, and a vitamin B complex would be a useful daily ancillary treatment.

Outcome:

Variable. Based on the level of poisoning. Presently, most exposures are mild and amenable to chelation. Development of a higher affinity chelator is necessary (stability > 18) to improve treatment and outcome.

Further Reading:

1.Zhao, B., Wang, Y., Li, X., & Wang, J. . Arsenic toxicity: sources, pathophysiology and mechanism. 2024. *Toxicological Research*, 13. Article.1093.

2.Cheng YF, Zhao Yj, Chen C Zhang F. Heavy Metal Toxicity: Mechanism, Health Effects, and Therapeutic Interventions. MedComm 2025; 6: 245-258.

3.Jaishankar M, Tseten T, Anbalagan N, Mathew BB, Beeregowda KN. Toxicity, mechanism and health effects of some heavy metals.Interdisciplinary Toxicology; 7: 60-72.

4. Martell AE, Smith RJ. authors.Title: Critical stability constants, Vol 6: Second Supplement. Plenum Press, NY, NY. 1992.

CHAPTER

Sixteen

RADIOACTIVE METALS. PLUTONIUM, URANIUM, CESIUM-13

Chapter 16. Radioactive metals. Plutonium, Uranium, Cesium-137

This chapter focuses on three of the most described radioactive metals regarding frequency and radiation toxicity. This chapter includes Cesium-137 which is radioactive. Stable Cesium is described in conjunction with Thallium, as these commonly occur together through oral consumption of affected produce.

When describing these heavy metals it is customary to include in their description the particular isotope (subtype/form), as the neutron number and atomic weight vary between them in addition to the half-life and level of radiation toxicity. This reflects that different isotopes often have different fissibility. Fissibility is defined as propensity to undergo radioactive decay with the release of energetic particles that cause radiation damage In other words the ability to undergo fission (splitting) of the atom.

The level of danger a radioactive metal possesses depends largely on two properties: 1) type of radiation emitted, and 2) the half life of decay, the shorter the half life the more dangerous.

Sources:

Plutonium:

1. Nuclear reactors. Nuclear fuel cycle.

Uranium:

1. More naturally occurring and much more plentiful than Plutonium. Uranium is found in rock, soil, and ground water.

2. Mining uranium ore.

3. Sites near prior nuclear weapons testing.

Cesium-137:

1. Nuclear weapons testing from mid-20th century.

2. Nuclear accidents, Chernobyl,Fukushima.

3. In the news in 2025, shrimp and cloves imported from Indonesia, presumed contamination from a nearby metal scrap-yard.

Who are at risk: Extent of exposure is the only demographic. A historic example of radium dial painters is watches and clocks. Sufferers would experience a high incidence of oral cancers, because they would lick the paint brush tips to make the point fine to paint the dials with radium.

Plutonium: Workers in nuclear facilities. Most radioactive metal workers fit this picture.

Uranium: Uranium has several isotopes. The two most common are U-235, which is the isotope that is described for nuclear weapons. and U-238 is the isotope that is found more naturally occurring. U-235 is more fissible and is an alpha particle emitter, which is the most damaging radiation emission. U-238 is the much more abundant isotope and is found naturally, U-238 is much more stable and persistent. This is the isotope found in the majority of individuals who have Uranium in their 24 hr urine specimens. Individuals living near sites where nuclear weapons testing occurred, in USA in south western locations, will have larger amounts of Uranium retained in their bodies.

Cesium:The 2025 finding of Cs- 137 contamination of shrimp and cloves from Indonesia, suggest that traditional sources for Cs-137, areas of nuclear bomb testing or nuclear power plant accidents, may now be expanding to include food items from various locations around the world.

Symptoms.

More than any other category of heavy metal toxicity, acute and chronic symptoms are distinct categories. Acute symptoms reflect the burning of tissues in closest contact with the radioactive metal exposure: so skin, eyes, and if inhaled lungs, and swallowed digestive tract. The most concerning Chronic toxicity is malignancy development: representing cancers arising from the sites of direct contact, and the most common malignancies are from cell types that are more radiosensitive: blood cell lines (example leukemia), thyroid, breast. Fibrosis/ scarring is a benign chronic finding, but can be very crippling. Typical sites of scarring are skin, lungs, digestive tract, eyes causing blindness, and joint contractures.

The larger the amount of highly destructive particle release with short half life, the more dangerous the radioactive metal. Essentially all isotopes of Plutonium are alpha particle emitters with comparatively shorter half life, so it is a very lethal radioactive metal. The isotopes of Uranium vary in the severity of potential injury, and the half-life is a common factor for the variability

Acute symptoms:

These vary in severity based on the dose, specific metal, and the exposure route.

1. Digestive tract issues. Nausea, vomiting, abdominal pain, diarrhea. (Ingestion)

2. Coughing, shortness of breath, chest pain (inhalation).

3. Rashes, redness, skin pain, skin sloughing. (skin exposure).

4. Headaches, dizziness, confusion, seizures, (neurological symptoms)

5. Fatigue, weakness, organ damage (liver, kidneys).(systemic symptoms).

6. Decreased vision.

Symptoms from the distant sites (neurological and systemic) reflect a combination of direct radioactive toxicity and immunological response (cytokine release, etc).

Chronic toxicity:

1. Malignancy is the chronic disease of greatest concern. Blood cell tumors, such as leukemia, are the most common and arise the earliest after exposure, generally with a delay of 2 years. Solid tumors onset more typically arise 10- 20 years post exposure. Breast, lung and thyroid cancers are three of the most common solid cancers. Since the exposure likely also entails inhalation of radioactive particles lung cancer and lung fibrosis are relatively common late onset diseases.

2. Fibrosis of skin, lungs, digestive tract.

Treatment:

Rapid initiation of chelation therapy is the essential treatment for radioactive metals. This is different for treatment of a stable heavy metal with abrupt exposure, such as Gd, because in this latter circumstance often some delay in initiating treatment to 3 months post exposure is employed, in order to see if the immune system calms down on its own. The difference is because the primary injury from radioactive metals is the deterministic effect of acute radiation damage, rather than the more variable and lesser harm of the immunological/ toxic injury from stable heavy metals. Accompaniment with steroid/ antihistamines is also appropriate with radioactive metals for similar, but at the same time somewhat distinct, reasons. For stable metals it is to control the immune response, whereas for radioactive metals it is to limit the damage from direct radiation toxicity primarily, with lesser consideration of controlling the host immune response.

The standard treatment for Plutonium has been daily iv Zn-DTPA treatment. DTPA stability is 22 with Plutonium. In earlier experience with cases of Plutonium release accidents in nuclear facilities, aerosolized delivery by masks had been used. This makes considerable empirical sense based on the type of exposure. Oral HOPO is also reported to have a stability constant of 22. Its use would be more broadly available to multiple individuals due to the ease of administration

Uranium is also treated with DTPA chelation although the stability constant is lower (stability 15) than it is for Plutonium (stability 22). HOPO has a similar stability for Uranium as DTPA, also stability 15.

We have described in an earlier chapter, that Ca-DTPA may be a better selection as it removes more heavy metal than Zn-DTPA. With perhaps 3 days of Ca-DTPA, one day native metal restitution, and repeating that cycle, as one type of regimen that makes empiric sense.

HOPO should also be effective for chelation. It has one advantage presently, as an oral agent it can more quickly be delivered to a broader population. My understanding is that HOPO has been used in various military scenarios, but results are unpublished and perhaps held as confidential information.

Cesium-137 is treated with oral Prussian Blue. Daily administration of 300 mg twice a day should be started immediately. Generally at least 1 month of daily Prussian Blue should be used.

Outcome:

There are three basic determinants of outcome: 1) the amount of radiation release by the radioactive metal, 2) the dose of the exposure, and 3) the speed of starting effective chelation.

Further Reading:

1 .Fukuda S. Chelating agents used for plutonium and uranium removal in radiation emergency medicine. Current Medicinal Chemistry 2005; 12: 2765-2770.

2. Martell AE, Smith RJ. authors.Title: Critical stability constants, Vol 6: Second Supplement. Plenum Press, NY, NY. 1992.

CHAPTER

Seventeen

THALLIUM AND CESIUM.

Chapter 17. Thallium and Cesium.

Thallium and stable Cesium are often elevated together on 24 hour urine samples. Both heavy metals can mimic Potassium in their uptake paths from soils.

Radioactive Cesium, CS-137, is a nuclear reactor byproduct and is included with the radioactive metals described in Chapter 16.

Sources:

Presently, the primary source for Thallium and Cesium are from cruciferous vegetables. These vegetables are noteworthy for picking up sulfur, but are also effective at picking up other nutrients and elements, such as Potassium.Thallium and to a lesser extent stable Cesium can mimic Potassium by uptake method, hence these toxic metals are efficiently taken up by these vegetables. By far the most efficient vegetable in taking them up is kale.

1.Kale, (Thallium, Cesium)

2. Ambient air and soil pollution (primarily vehicle emissions) (Thallium, Cesium)..

3. Metal smelting (Thallium)
4. Electronic waste (Thallium)
5. Historic rodenticide (Thallium)

Thallium is infamous as a nefarious poison since it was readily available as a rat poison (no longer) and is difficult to detect in the corpse.

Who are at risk: Most of the reports of Thallium toxicity have been in white women. It is not clear if this reflects a lifestyle dietary cause (excess consumption of kale) or if there is also a genetic cause. White women in general are more susceptible to many Immune Mediated Inflammatory Diseases (IMID). Likely the dominant explanation is dietary choices.

Symptoms:

1. Fatigue, weakness.
2. Hair loss.
3. Neurological: Peripheral numbness and tingling (hands and feet).
4. Digestive Tract: Nausea. Abdominal pain.
5. In severe cases central nervous system symptoms of confusion and coordination problems.

Avoidance:

The simplest and first method to manage Thallium and Cesium is to stop eating kale entirely. The person must replace kale with the least heavy metal concentrating cruciferous vegetable which is broccoli.

Detoxification:

Standard nonspecific methods of detoxification, with the principle most critical addition of abstaining from eating Kale.

Treatment.

Oral Prussian Blue. Recommend 1 g orally 3 times per day to start. This can be increased to 3 g orally 3 times per day. This agent has high binding affinity in the gut for Thallium and Cesium.

Prussian Blue behaves differently from other chelators in that it stays in the intestines. The mechanism is different in that it has a lattice structure that can trap certain cations (positively charged particles) which includes Thallium and Cesium. Prussian Blue behaves like a molecular trap in the small intestine, it serves as a molecular cage and prevents re-absorption into the body through the small intestine.

Although Thallium and Cesium act systemically, the removal with Prussian Blue acts solely through the gut. This occurs as follows:Thallium and Cesium both undergo hepatobiliary excretion as the natural form of elimination. In the natural state a certain percentage of the Thallium and Cesium excreted in bile gets re-absorbed back through the small intestine into the blood circulation. A sizable percentage of these metals experience a circular pathway. Prussian Blue acts to break the circular pathway of maintaining Thallium and Cesium in the body..

A fair amount of these metals are also eliminated by the kidneys, hence 24 hr urine is an effective tool to identify an excess presence of these metals. There is a dual elimination pathway for these metals by kidneys and hepatobiliary, the relative proportions may be around 50/50.

Stool sampling would be an ideal method for testing both the presence of Thallium and Cesium and the elimination by Prussian Blue. In general I have not been fond of stool sampling, not only from the concept, but also the motility of the digestive tract has a far more variable timeline than renal elimination.

The binding affinity for Thallium and Cesium is only fair with DMSA, EDTA, and DTPA, in the 8-10 range. So they are not optimal.

Agents such as HOPO that have dual renal and hepatobiliary elimination may be an effective ancillary chelation means to remove these metals. To date this is untested.

Outcome:

Stopping consumption of Kale, and in some severe cases, using Prussian Blue should result in a very good outcome for the majority of sufferers.

Further Reading::

1.Thompson JR, Evans ML, Williams SK, et al. Management of Thallium and Cesium Poisoning: A Comprehensive Review.Clinical toxicology. 2021; 59: 289-302.

CHAPTER

Eighteen

BERYLLIUM.

Chapter 18. Beryllium.

Beryllium is a lighter weight, not a heavy metal. It is in the alkaline earth metal group, which also includes Magnesium and Calcium. Several aspects of Beryllium toxicity are interesting and worth describing on its own

Sources:

1. Beryllium is a lightweight yet strong heavy metal so has broad industrial use.
2. Manufacturing of aerospace components, electronics, metallurgy.
3. Janitorial work in plants working with Beryllium

Who are at risk: Individuals who inhale dust particles of Beryllium..

Symptoms:

Beryllium toxicity is primarily centered on the lungs arising from inhalation of dust created from manufacturing processes directly or in clean-up. Chronic toxicity from Beryllium is termed Chronic Beryllium Disease (CBD). This could also be called Beryllium Deposition Disease.

1. Acute Beryllium exposure results in a picture of persistent coughing, due to irritation of the bronchi, bronchioles and alveoli. The greater the volume of exposure the greater the severity of coughing.

2. Chronic Beryllium exposure:

CBD- chronic disease. Acute disease may lead to CBD based on the length of time of exposure and volume of exposure. This results in an interstitial lung disease. The symptoms are chronic cough and as the interstitial lung disease advances, progressively severe dyspnea (inability to breathe) develop,

Avoidance: If there is suspicion of acute Beryllium exposure symptoms, the primary treatment is removal of the individual from that work place environment.

Detoxification/ Treatment: The primary treatment has been the use of immune reaction suppressing drugs.

1. Steroids. Standard treatment.
2. More potent immune modulating drugs. rapamycin, methotrexate, azathioprine. I may prefer low dose rapamycin.
3. Chelation has not been used for treatment.
4. Bronchopulmonary lavage has been used as part of the diagnostic tools to diagnose CBD. Its use for treatment though has not been established, but empirically it sounds reasonable, especially with steroid containing normal saline lavage.

Discussion:

Beryllium is useful to describe separately from other lighter weight metals that can cause toxicity (such as Aluminum) because Beryllium can cause a much more intense immunological response. This reflects the underlying chemistry of Beryllium and its interaction with the host. Beryllium can bond with certain host proteins and that complex results in a profound immunological response.

One important aspect of this immunological response is that a test has been developed to look for CBD, by detecting the immune system reaction to the presence of Beryllium. This test is termed the Beryllium lymphocyte proliferation test or BeLPT. This involves: blood sampling, and extracting lymphocytes from the sample. This starts with centrifugation to isolate the white blood cells and then more refined separation to isolate lymphocytes, such as density gradient or use of special media. The isolated lymphocytes then are exposed to Beryllium in solution to examine for lymphocyte reaction and proliferation.

A similar concept has been used to look for the potential of GBCAs to result in an acute hypersensitivity reaction (AHR) with a pin prick technique. Individual MR GBCAs are injected as tiny (1 ml) amounts of intradermally to evaluate for the development of an immune reaction. This is not commonly performed, and I am uncertain of its level of accuracy. It would seem that a Lymphocyte Proliferation Test may be a more accurate method to look for the immunological component of Gd and other heavy metals toxicities. I am not aware if this has been done. The importance of describing Beryllium in this book is that it is relatively unique as an almost pure inhalational metal toxicity and because of the use of the BeLPT, an immunologic stimulation test to detect disease.The development of the test for other heavy metals seems worth investigating.

The established recognition of the prominent immunological role of the toxicity with Beryllium, provides insight into the importance of immunological response for all heavy metals. Likely the risk of CBD from exposure is similar to the risks for most other heavy metals: 1 in 10,000 individuals exposed to the metal may have the immune system factors that create the propensity for the disease.

Finally, as CBD is an inhalational form of interstitial lung disease, as with other inhalational lung diseases, such as smoke inhalation, it is predominantly an upper lobe interstitial lung disease

Outcome: Once the disease has progressed to CBD and if the amount of toxin has been large, management of the interstitial lung disease by immune dampening drugs has only fair outcome at best, managing rather than curing disease. Early recognition of acute exposure and avoiding further workplace exposure would result in an excellent outcome.

Further Reading:

1.MacMurdo MG, Mroz MM, CulverDA, Dweik RA, Maier LA. Chronic Beryllium Disease: Update on a Moving Target. 2020. Chest ;158: 2458-2466.

2. Elguero J, Alkorta I. The Dubious Origin of Beryllium Toxicity.Structural Chemistry; 34: 391=398.

CHAPTER

Nineteen

CHROMIUM.

Chapter 19. Chromium.

Chromium is relatively unique among heavy metals in that it is also an element that is part of the normal functioning of human physiology. There are two forms, trivalent Chromium which takes part in normal physiology and hexavalent Chromium which is toxic.Trivalent Chromium is involved in the body handling of insulin and sugar.

Sources Hexavalent Chromium:

1. Manufacturing and metal working: chrome plating, stainless steel production, chrome based pigments.
2. Contaminated soil and water from industrial run-off.

Noteworthy is that Erin Brokovich began her efforts against pollution and toxins from her initial work identifying hexavalent Chromium as the responsible toxin in a community that suffered from severe toxicity from industrial run-off.

Who are at risk: Individuals with high exposure to hexavalent Chromium.

Symptoms:

1. Irritation of the nose, throat and lungs from inhalation.
2. Dermatitis and skin ulceration.
3. Nasal and sinus issues. Nose bleeds.
4. Digestive tract reactions: nausea, vomiting, diarrhea, abdominal pain.
5. Kidney and liver damage.
6. Malignancy development. Lung cancer, gastrointestinal cancers, leukemia, lymphoma (chronic).

Avoidance: If symptoms develop for hexavalent Chromium toxicity, and you are employed in the above described work environments, cease working there.

Detoxification: Standard detoxification with the critical addition of **vitamin C and alpha-lipoic acid** (below).

Treatment:

Chromium is nearly unique among the heavy metals in that chelation is not the primary therapy. In large part because trivalent chromium is part of normal human physiology and depleting this with chelation would result in significant health issues such as diabetes.

Therefore the primary approach is the chemical reaction of reduction of hexavalent Chromium to trivalent Chromium. This is achieved with acidic oral agents. The gentlest of which is ascorbic acid, vitamin C. The addition of another anti-oxidant alpha-lipoic acid is also used in combination with vitamin C.

Standard regimen: Vitamin C 1 - 2 g daily with alpha-lipoic acid 0.3 to 0.6 g daily.

It should however be noted that the stability constants are very high with Chromium for both EDTA (23-25) and DTPA (26-28) so they would be very effective at removing Chromium. In individuals with high exposure to hexavalent Chromium, an appropriate treatment regimen would also include careful use of EDTA or DTPA chelation.

Caution: Note that a common ancillary therapy tried for many of the Immune Mediated Inflammatory Disorders (IMIDs) and other similar disorders is Hyperbaric Oxygen Therapy (HBOT). Oxygenation shows benefit for many disorders, among them traumatic brain injury. Since HBOT increases oxygen it will drive the reaction from trivalent Chromium to hexavalent Chromium, so this is contra-indicated for Chromium toxicity, because it likely will increase the extent of toxicity.

Outcome: Variable, depending on severity of disease.

Further Reading:

1.Shin DY, Lee SM, Jang Y, et al. Adverse Human Health Effects of Chromium by Exposure Route: A Comprehensive Review Based on Toxicogenomic Approach. 2023; International Journal of Molecular Science. 24:3410-3418.:

CHAPTER

Twenty

PLATINUM AND PALLADIUM

Chapter 20. Platinum and Palladium

Palladium, platinum, rhodium, ruthenium. iridium and osmium are members of a group of elements referred to as the platinum group metals. They share similar chemical properties,

Sources:

Platinum is a common metal used in chemotherapy drugs: cisplatin, carboplatin, and oxaliplatin. Toxicity for these is related to the drug in its entirety and not to Platinum as an element.

Elemental Platinum and Palladium are used in catalytic converters. Factory workers in electronics and catalytic converter manufacture, and may show up in 24 hr urine in individuals studied for other metals.

A small quantity of Platinum and Palladium are present in dental amalgams.

Who are at risk: exposure dose. Platinum-containing oncology drugs hypersensitivity may also have genetic factors. Note this hypersensitivity is to the entirety of the drug, and not to elemental Platinum.

Symptoms:

Platinum: Platinum, like Gd, has a role in medical practice. Also like Gd, Platinum-based chemotherapy agents are administered as iv injections, and therefore result in a more abrupt intravascular exposure. This may explain why Acute Hypersensitivity Reactions (AHR) are recognized for both Platinum oncology drugs and Gd, but not a significant adverse event for other heavy metals, whose incorporation is oral and therefore more protracted and insidious. Note that in the case of Platinum the AHR is a reaction to the entire drug, and not to elemental Platinum *per se.* Platinum-containing cancer drugs are administered as long iv infusions, whereas GBCAs are administered as rapid bolus injections.

Acute Hypersensitivity reactions:

1. skin rash
2. respiratory distress
3. Anaphylaxis.

Some of the acute reactions are IgE-mediated.

Chronic reactions:

Unlike with GBCAs, where the symptom profile is similar if not identical between all brands of GBCAs, the toxicities of each platinum chemotherapy compound is different. With Gd, it supports the theory that the reaction is to the Gd element, whereas with the Platinum cancer drugs the reaction may be to the compound in its entirety, including Platinum, but not to Platinum itself per se. The different toxicities of the Platinum agents are as follows: for cisplatin nephrotoxicity, carboplatin causes more severe myelosuppression but is less nephrotoxic. Oxaliplatin exhibits unique acute neurotoxicity and cumulative sensory neurotoxicity, observed following ongoing treatment. A treatment approach termed rapid desensitization has shown notable success, involving the careful and controlled administration of incrementally increasing doses under close supervision.

Specific toxicity to elemental Platinum and Palladium has not been well described, and if it occurs presently it is very rare.

Avoidance: In the event that chemotherapy drugs cause a severe reaction, the approaches used are switching to another Platinum containing drug, or switching to another category of chemotherapy altogether.

Detoxification: Standard detoxification, with including specific attention to the chemotherapeutic agent.

Treatment:

Chemotherapy based Platinum.

Acute Hypersensitivity Reactions:

1. Steroids and antihistamines. Both in the setting of Premedication and Post- symptom development.

Chronic Symptoms:

1. Nephrotoxicity can be minimized by adequate hydration prior to treatment.
2. Prolonging infusion administration.
3. Rapid desensitization regimens, which involves controlled incremental dose escalation in sequential treatment sessions.

No specific treatment for elemental Platinum or Palladium.

Stability constants Platinum and Palladium: DMSA (12), EDTA (18-19), DTPA (21).The reactions to these Platinum based cancer drugs are due to the entire drug and not Platinum, so chelation not indicated.

Outcomes:

The reactions to Platinum-based chemotherapeutic agents are a reaction to the entire agent, and not to elemental Platinum. So this strictly speaking is not a Platinum toxicity reaction. The inclusion in this book is to illustrate that point for a particular heavy metal. In depth discussion of Platinum-based cancer drugs is not made, because the reactions relate to the cancer drug as a whole.

Elemental Platinum and Palladium are to date not recognized as appreciably toxic. Based on stability constants DTPA shows the highest affinity for these metals.

Further Reading::

1.Feng G, Zhou X, Chen J,Li D, Chen L.Platinum Drugs-related Safety Profile: The Latest Five-year Analysis from FDA Adverse Event Reporting System Data. 2023. Frontiers in Oncology. 12: article 1012093.

CHAPTER

Twenty One

METAL TOXICITY FROM LOWER ATOMIC NUMBER METALS.

Chapter 21. Management of metal toxicity from lower atomic number metals: Iron, Copper, Aluminum, Nickel.

Essential metals vs nonessential (foreign) metals.

Lower atomic number (lighter weight) metals that are considered essential (necessary for life) include: Iron (Fe), Copper (Cu), Magnesium (Mg), Manganese (Mn), Calcium (Ca), and Potassium (K). Note we often do not think of Ca and K as metals, but they are.

Lower atomic number (lighter weight) nonessential metals include: Aluminum, Nickel, Thallium (in an earlier chapter), Beryllium (in an earlier chapter), Antimony and Tin.

Treatment of essential metals depends on whether there is deficiency, a situation in which supplementation is needed, or excessive, in which detoxification or removal is necessary. Since essential metals are necessary for life, removal has to be done with care not to remove too much. This work focuses on removal of toxicity.In contrast, nonessential removal does not have the constraint of concern over removing too much.

Excess iron.

The most common excessive state of essential metals is excessive Iron, and the most common condition that is toxic is Genetic Hemochromatosis (GH).Overall transfusion-related excess iron (transfusional siderosis) is a much more common form of iron overload, but is rarely toxic.

S**ource**: GH is a genetic disease that reflects increased absorption of Iron from the digestive tract.

Symptoms: The adverse health impact of the excess intracorporeal iron is on the pancreas (resulting in pancreatic insufficiency), the liver (liver failure, hepatocellular cancer), heart (heart failure), If untreated, death usually results from heart failure, liver cirrhosis, or hepatocellular cancer

Who are at risk: White people of Gaulic (French) origin. HFE gene, most often C282Y mutation.

Treatment:

1. Phlebotomy (blood letting). Early detection and early treatment may be sufficient management.

2. Chelation. Deferoxamine. For more advanced deposition.Regimen: 20-40 mg/ kg per day given as a slow iv injection over 8 - 12 hours, 4 times/ week.

Outcome: excellent with early detection and treatment.

Copper overload. Wilson's Disease.

Source: Decreased ability of the liver to excrete Copper into the bile, resulting in intracorporeal build up of Copper.

Symptoms:

The build up of Copper has the greatest impact on the liver and neurological system.

1. The distinctive clinical feature is the Kayser-Fleischer Ring, a coppery,

golden-brown ring around the cornea.

2. Tremors, decreased coordination, speech alteration, mood and personality changes, depression.

3. Liver failure. Fatigue. Jaundice.

Who is at risk: Autosomal recessive disease affecting the ATP7B gene. No gender or racial predilection.

Treatment:

Chelation with penicillamine. Penicillamine forms a coordinate bond with Copper, which renders it water-soluble and excretable through urine. The regimen is oral Penicillamine 250 mg - 500 mg two to four times per day, generally starting at a lower amount then building up. Treatment is usually lifelong.

Outcome:

If detected early and treated the outcome is very good.

Aluminum Toxicity:

Sources: Patients on hemodialysis, from the dialysate fluid or aluminum-containing phosphate binders. Current dialysis care has largely eliminated these impurities. Aluminum workers. Factory workers involved with aluminum-containing products, such as cars. Exposure to aluminum dust. Aluminum in cookware. Aluminum-containing antacids. Aluminum-containing antiperspirants.

The greatest exposures are with hemodialysis patients and factory workers.

Symptoms:

1. Neurological symptoms: the greatest concern with aluminum is its potential to cause various forms of dementia.

2. Bone deposition. Bone pain. Osteomalacia.

3. Kidney failure.

Who are at risk: Renal dialysis patients. Aluminum factory workers.

Avoidance: If high levels of aluminum are present in native 24 hr urine, the individual should be removed from the work environment if the source is occupational.

Treatment:

Chelation with deferoxamine. For dialysis patients administration is tailored to the dialysis schedule. Typical dose 5mg/ kg given over the last hour of dialysis, a few times per week.

Outcome:

If detected early and treated early the outcome is fair in individuals who are already symptomatic.

Nickel:

The most common reaction to nickel is a topical allergic response to Nickel, and this generally is due to Nickel-containing jewelry. Nickel also can be a systemic disease. This is described below:

Sources:

1. Nickel-containing jewelry.
2. Occupational exposure.
3. Medical implants
4. Nickel-containing foods.

Symptoms:

1. widespread dermatitis or eczema.
2. respiratory asthma-type symptoms. Chronic cough.
3. chronic fatigue. Generalized malaise.
4. Headache
5. Joint pain.

Who are at risk: Factory workers in Nickel industry.

Retention location: This depends on how the metal exposure occurred. As skin is a common site, then skin is the largest reservoir. If the exposure is through inhalation of dust, then lungs would be a prominent site. Some nickel is also retained in kidneys, liver, and brain.

Avoidance: Avoid nickel containing jewelry and other nickel products if topical reaction is the source. .Stop work in Nickel factory work if respiratory origin..

Detoxification: General detoxification.

Treatment:

1. Skin lesions can be treated with topical steroids.

2. Systemic disease can benefit from steroids to decrease inflammation, and chelation to remove the metal. The stability constants are as follows: DMSA (8-10), EDTA (10-11), DTPA (12). None of the chelators show high affinity (20 reflects high affinity and a very good chelator) so chelation is not as effective as for most heavy metals. Of the 3, DTPA has the highest stability and hence is preferred.

Outcome: None of the chelators are that effective at removing Nickel so outcome often reflects chronicity and total body content.

Further Reading:

1. Adams PC, Ryanz JD, Diagnosis and Treatment of Hemochromatosis.2025. Narrative Reviews; 23:issue 9p1477.

2. Rodriguez-Castro KI; Hevia-Urrutia FJ, Sturniolo C.Wilson's Disease: A Review of What We Have Learned.2015. World Journal of Hepatology; 7: 2859-2870.

3. Igbokwe IO, Igwenagu E, Igbokwe NA. Aluminum Toxicosis: a Review of Toxic Actions and Effects.2020. Interdisciplinary Toxicology; 12: 45-70.

4.Genchi G, Carocci A, Lauria G, Sinicropi MS, Catalano A. Nickel: Human Health and Environmental Toxicology. 2020. Nickel: Human Health and Environmental Toxicology. 17: 679-691

CHAPTER

Twenty Two

FINAL THOUGHTS

Chapter 22. Final Thoughts.

The intention of this book is to provide succinct practical information on the toxicity and treatment of multiple heavy metals. The cellular and metabolic interferences created by the various metals are fascinating and also remarkable for the complex forms of damages that they each create.

In a textbook intended for a knowledgeable general audience, the chemistry does not fundamentally add practical information, and describing the details of chemical injury may be overwhelming for the reader to process and distract from the key points. This would take away the focus of the principle intention: who are at risk, what are the symptoms, and what is the current most effective treatment that individuals should undergo. The focus therefore has been on the most current and effective therapy to treat the toxicity caused by a variety of heavy metals. The reader is now armed with the knowledge of what should be performed to treat a full array of heavy metals. If the reader has a heavy metal toxicity, they now know what they should receive. I have written exactly what our regimens are, as the major chelation center in the world. In fact I anticipate patients should use the regimens in this book to instruct their physicians what they should be receiving, and if they cannot get the treatment locally, they can go elsewhere to get treatment, including to our clinic.

This book clears up the misapprehension that many allopathic physicians may have that there is no science to chelation and it may be quackery. I have outlined the features of science which are as solid as for any other disease process. The foundation for treatment is understanding the composite of the highest stability constant chelator available combined with lab evidence that it is working in the individual, focusing on 24 hr urine measurements. When to start and when to stop has also been addressed. The other critical observation is to be aware that heavy metal toxicity is a two-hit mechanism of 1) dysfunctioning of the immune system, which allows 2) the intrinsic toxicity of the metal to manifest, creating the overall picture of effective toxicity. So both immune system damage and metal toxicity need to be addressed.

For the future, an anticipated new edition would be based on when new more effective and more readily accessible chelators are available. In the short term future, I am focused on oral forms of high stability chelators with broad coverage. At that time, as with this edition, the focus will be on a practical effective treatment regimen.

www.ingramcontent.com/pod-product-compliance
Lightning Source LLC
LaVergne TN
LVHW022220200926
848481LV00006B/2046
* 9 7 9 8 2 1 8 8 6 1 9 1 9 *